The International Library of Psychology

NERVOUS DISORDERS AND CHARACTER

Founded by C. K. Ogden

The International Library of Psychology

GENERAL PSYCHOLOGY
In 38 Volumes

NERVOUS DISORDERS AND CHARACTER

A Study in Pastoral Psychology and Psychotherapy

JOHN G McKENZIE

First published in 1946 by
Routledge and Kegan Paul Ltd

Reprinted in 1999 by
Routledge
2 Park Square, Milton Park, Abingdon, Oxon, OX14 4RN

Transferred to Digital Printing 2006

Routledge is an imprint of the Taylor & Francis Group

© 1946 John G McKenzie

British Library Cataloguing in Publication Data
A CIP catalogue record for this book
is available from the British Library

Nervous Disorders and Character
ISBN 978-0415-21033-1
General Psychology: 38 Volumes
ISBN 0415-21129-8
The International Library of Psychology: 204 Volumes
ISBN 0415-19132-7
Printed and bound by CPI Antony Rowe, Eastbourne

PREFACE

My first word must be one of thanks to the Principal and Governors of Manchester College, Oxford, for the honour and opportunity of delivering the series of Tate Lectures which constitute the substance of this small volume. The hospitality, so charmingly dispensed by the Principal's wife, Mrs. Cross, is a happy memory which I share with many officers of the army whose duties took them to Oxford in wartime. Nor shall I soon forget the thoughtful kindnesses of the Principal, the keen discussions of the students in the Common Room in the evenings, all of which added to the enjoyment of my visits. I was greatly privileged to take the services in the College Chapel and to preside at the Sacrament of the Lord's Supper.

The Lectures themselves are almost as delivered except for an enlargement here and there, and for the omission of some illustrations which, although they would have added to the value of the volume, could not be inserted because the subject of the illustration might have been recognized. They embody some of the conclusions I have reached in regard to the relation between Nervous Disorders and Character-structure. In another series, to be delivered in 1947 in Manchester College, I hope to deal specifically with the Religious Factor in these disorders. In addition to showing the personality-factor in nervous troubles I have outlined what I think is the sphere of Pastoral Psychology in relation to Psychotherapy and Psychopathology. In the final lecture there will be found the situation which gives rise to the symptoms, hints about mental hygiene, a characterization

v

of the mature adult, and a word as to what the pastor can do. I have also, in the third lecture, described various mental processes such as the "unconscious motive", repression and rationalization which are still imperfectly understood even by distinguished writers in philosophy and religion.

In thirty years' study of the neuroses, and twenty-five years of personal dealing with the victims of neurotic conflict, one's attitude changes as deeper insight into the character of both the conflicts and their causes develops. I believe, in contrast to Freud and the Psycho-analytical school, that not the "external factor" in the causation of neurotic conflict is the most important, but the internal factor, namely, the individual's moral and religious character. And I believe also that a change in the latter alone can constitute a "cure".

As far as I know, I have given references to the authors quoted. That, however, is not the extent of my indebtedness to others. I am debtor to all schools of psychology, but I am more indebted to my patients. I would specially make mention of the writings of Erich Fromm and Karen Horney. They have helped me to crystallize trends of thought of which I have been conscious for some years. I believe their approach from the side of personality instead of from the side of "repressed complexes" is the way to real progress in psychology and psychotherapy. There is need for a deeper study of the personality as a whole, as a dynamic unity, from the psychological point of view.

Many people have been disappointed at not being able to purchase a copy of my *Souls in the Making*. It has been for some time out of print. It needs to be re-written throughout to fulfil the purpose of a true Introduction to Pastoral Psychology. I hope, however, that this small volume will meet the need for such an introduction to a subject of increasing importance to all who have to deal with the personal problems of our time.

My thanks are due to Rev. H. Newsham, M.A., Edinburgh, for the careful reading of the MS. in type, and the suggestions he made. To my daughter, Dr. Margaret R. Laws, M.A., and her husband, Dr. F. Laws, I am grateful for their careful correction of the proofs.

Paton College,
  Nottingham, 1946.

CONTENTS

CHARACTER-STRUCTURE
AND PERSONALITY-DISORDERS

THE passing of the Education Bill is not the only sign of a growing consciousness that the curricula of Educational Bodies must be overhauled if we are to meet the complicated problems of both society and the individual in the post-war years. The Royal College of Physicians has issued its report on the training of medical students ; and one of the points it emphasizes in its recommendations is that there must be given to every prospective doctor a more rational education in psychological medicine. Not only should the medical practitioner be able to diagnose organic disease, but he must be able to recognize and treat if possible, or refer to the specialist, disorders whose causative factors lie in the mind and character of the patient.

It is a common-place that an individual may be sound in every organ of his body and yet manifest physical symptoms of a distressing kind, such as heart disturbance, disorders of the alimentary canal, functional paralysis, debilitating headaches, excessive fatigue. Indeed, there seems to be few organic diseases which the neurotic individual cannot unconsciously simulate. On the other hand, there may be no sign of physical symptoms, but the patient may complain of disturbed sleep in which he wakens full of anxiety, apprehensiveness, and covered with perspiration ; or he confesses to irrational fears which make his life a torture : the fear of closed places ; of going out alone ; of crossing the street ; of going insane ; of violent feelings accompanied by the fear of doing bodily harm to someone ; a fear of suffering from some particular disease such as syphilis or cancer. These are but a few of the fears of which patients complain ; and which, through a more rational education in psychological medicine, the practitioner will at least understand even if he cannot undertake treatment himself.

Untrained in psychology the doctor is apt to put these symptoms down to imagination, and counsel the patient to pull himself together. He may tell his patient that " it is all nerves ", and try to bully him out of the trouble. Medicine is now to be told that there is no such thing as imaginary pain ; if a patient thinks he has pain, he has pain ; if a patient is full of fear he is afraid. We cannot imagine we are afraid ; imagination in its attempt to explain the fear may ascribe it to an object of which there is no need to be afraid ; or imagination can exaggerate the fearsomeness of an object, but it cannot create the fear. The doctor is right in telling his patient that there is no organic basis for his pain or that his fear is irrational, but that leaves the subjective causes of the pain or fear to be investigated.

Many of the disturbances of which the patient complains are in the realm of character ; and the doctor is not seldom called to give a report to a court of justice in regard to moral aberrations. The great majority of the patients suffering from character-disturbance or " nerves " complain of feelings of guilt, and in many of the anxiety—and depression—states. the sense of guilt and fear of God are marked symptoms. So marked is this symptom that Stekel went so far as to say that every neurotic suffers from a guilty conscience.[1]

Is it to be wondered at that the medical practitioner with little or no psychological training is bewildered and even impatient when he finds people complaining of aches and pains, fears and feelings, which have no organic basis ? The very fact that he advises them to " pull themselves together " shows that he thinks it is the will that needs

[1] *Conditions of Nervous Anxiety and Their Treatment*, page 22.

strengthening rather than the body. When he tells them " it is all nerves " he is dimly conscious of the fact that something is disturbing the normal function of the nerves. Doubtless he ought to have seen and acknowledged that the patient's disease was that he could not pull himself together ; and he ought to have been able to diagnose a disturbance of emotions ; but how can we blame him if his whole training has been limited to a study of disease of an organic kind ? How was it possible for him to detect the causes of rebellion in a son, or the delinquencies of a daughter ? What training in pathology could help a man to see that his patient was suffering from an envy which had become pathological, or that repressed pride was the reason why the patient could not bend his back, or that his suffering was spiritual and his disease was one of the soul and will ? If there is half a truth in the wide generalization of Dr. Jung that " A psycho-neurosis must be understood as the suffering of a human being who has not discovered what life means to him,"[1] then it follows that the medical practitioner " is not obliged to deal with it ". As Dr. Jung notes, the practitioner " is not obliged to have a finished outlook on life, and his professional conscience does not demand it of him ".[2] If, to paraphrase Dr. Jung,[3] a man is suffering from an inability to love, or because he has no faith he is afraid to grope in the dark, or is without hope because the world has disillusioned him ; and if he is suffering because life has lost its meaning for him, what can the doctor be expected to do ? These ills are due to the lack of the graces, the theological virtues, as the Fathers called them. They are conveyed by him that " bringeth good tidings ", whose feet are " shod with the Gospel of peace " and by nothing that the doctor can bring from his pharmacy.

[1] *Modern Man in Search of a Soul*, page 260.
[2] Ibid., page 260.
[3] Ibid., page 260.

3

From all this it can be inferred that neurotic disturbances of the personality are intimately connected with character-structure, our spiritual outlook on life, and our ethical ideals. If that is granted, then the Church cannot stand aloof. Indeed, the tragedy of the present-day Church is that she has failed to give the community a meaning to life. He reads the signs of the times wrongly who translates the failure of the Church in terms of our disturbed national and international relations, or in its failure to prevent war, or in our distorted social order. Social order is always the product of personality, the expression of what life means to a particular community, the values a community seeks to realize. If our social order is distorted, if gross inequalities of opportunity exist, if blatant wealth, and soul-destroying poverty live on opposite sides of the same streets, then it is because the Church has failed in one of its main tasks, namely, to socialize the individual. To evangelize is to socialize ; to evangelize is to give to the individual a meaning to life, and a relation to God, it is to make him capable of faith, hope, love and insight. Our social order is the creation of individuals ; it is sustained by the energy and aims of individuals. The modern world, with its dictators and totalitarian forms of government, illustrates the dictum of Carlyle that the history of a nation is just the biographies of its leading individuals. It is true that once a social order is created it has an objective existence and begins to shape the individual. We must be careful, however, to realize what that means. It does not mean that the social order is a living thing that exerts an irresistible power upon individuals. No ! *We are shaped by the social order in the sense that we have to fit ourselves into it.* When a social order is changed it is because some individual challenged its assumptions, refused to fit into it ; and thus a movement for change was instituted.

That is why the Gospel seems to have so little to say to

4

society as such. Christ deals with that which produces the social order, that which creates or changes a social order—the individual. Society is the product of personality, and personality is always individual ; there is no such thing as a group personality.

Hence the problem of society, if we think in ultimate terms, is the problem of Character : its formation ; its disturbances ; its perversions. Personality, as we shall see later, has as one of its most determining factors, the individual's religion or philosophy of life. If the giving of that is not the great function of the Church, what is ? Thus the Church cannot stand aside from the problems of neuroticism. Ministers are more involved here than the doctor. If medical training is to insist that medical students must be trained to recognize character-structure as a cause of the many troubles brought to the surgery ; if they are to be taught through an education in psychology to recognize the difference between an organic disease and diseases of the will, surely the Church has an obligation to see that the candidates for the ministry will have a rational training in that science which is most intimately connected with character-formation, namely psychology. Just as theology has always used the implications of philosophical theory if they would help her to ground and validate her beliefs, so the Church must learn from psychopathology and psychotherapy as well as from general psychology if she is to understand the spiritual diseases of her children ; and from them she must learn their need of true spiritual direction.

Our position is that the psychoneuroses are the outcome of character-disturbance ; that maladjustments to life, or the failure to adjust to life, the disturbance of the " nerves " which prevents the individual from being able to " pull himself together ", the thousand and one symptoms which have their origin in the mind, have their roots in character-defect ; and that if they are to be prevented or complete cure to be effected the development of a religious character is a necessity. We shall see later that there are many disturbances of character which are due to constitutional or organic causes. Meantime, let us turn to the study of facts rather than theories.

How close is the connection between the psychoneuroses and training in religious character can be seen in the observation of Dr. Jung. He says " he has never seen a patient in the second half of life whose trouble was not due in the last resort to the fact that he never had or had lost that which religion gives to all her devotees ".[1] Nor, he adds, has he ever seen one cured who did not regain or find religion.

That observation, I should think, most psychotherapists could confirm in their own practice. In over twenty years' experience of these disorders, I can truly say that, in a large number of cases, I have seen the symptoms disappear. But the disappearance of the symptoms is not a cure, as Freud himself testified. I have seen the symptoms disappear and little sign of them has been conscious to the patient, and yet after a certain time a return of the symptoms has been experienced, and indeed in an intensified form. The oversimplified idea that these troubles were due to some complex that had just to be brought to consciousness for the symptoms to evaporate has long been exploded. There are disturbances which are due to a failure to meet some particular situation, or to the attempt to repress a physiological drive like sex, or to a frustration of sex, and such will yield, sometimes with difficulty, to psychotherapeutic treatment, and give no further trouble ; but the neuroses in which the personality becomes distorted and which manifest themselves in distressing symptoms are invariably due to some neurotic trend whose roots lie in character-structure. The attempt to control masturbation by repression instead of by self-control will produce such

[1] Ibid., page 264.

a disturbance ; the frustration entailed by the death of the marriage partner often causes such a disturbance ; an experience whose memory has been repressed and which has become active in the unconscious may bring guilt-feelings for which no cause can be found in the patient's present life. Not a few of this kind of disturbance are due to wrong methods of birth-control or to repressed scruples in regard to it, and they may be cleared up without any deep change of character. But those disturbances of personality which are accompanied by the more distressing symptoms of neurotic disease, or through which the individual is maladjusted to life require for their cure a drastic change in the individual's whole outlook on life. These latter are what Karen Horney has called *character-neuroses*.[1]

Many of the people who consult the psychologist to-day do not suffer from any of the symptoms which are generally associated with a neurosis. They are not depressed ; they have no fears. Yet they are conscious that life has not a compelling interest for them ; they are awkward in their relations with other people ; if they make friends they choose the wrong people ; they are regular attenders at Church, but even if they are not bored they seem to get nothing from their worship. We have people consulting us because they are conscious that they are unable to fall in love, or if they do they at once become panicky immediately they get engaged and the engagement has to be broken off. There are others who seem incapable of making decisions or of having an opinion of their own. We have seen people who have been tireless in public work or in Church ; they became conscious that their many activities were motivated not by the cause they were serving, but by inward compulsions which kept them incapable of relaxation. The number of married people whose relations are strained, who nag each other from morn-

---

[1] *The Neurotic Personality of Our Time,* Chapter I.

7

ing to night, who are continually looking for faults in each other, who threaten once or twice a week to separate, must really be far greater than the outsider can imagine. All these people carry on with their usual duties and suffer no disabling symptoms. Nevertheless, they are conscious that from the point of view of happiness, character and personality they have failed miserably. They are often torn between love and hostile feelings directed towards the same person ; they are hot and cold towards the same interest or cause ; they feel drawn to religion yet find themselves cynical regarding it. Their interior life is at sixes and sevens ; it is ununified ; it is not disintegrated, but unintegrated ; their character is not closely knit together. It is these manifestations of character with which the psychotherapist has to deal ; and until these are thoroughly understood we shall not understand neuroticism even of the less distressing types.

Freud, to whom every psychologist owes his first insight into neurotic disease and character disturbance, was attracted by the manifestations of the erotic tendencies. To the frustration of these tendencies he traced the immediate causes of psychological abnormalities. " The most immediate," he writes, " most easily discerned, and most comprehensible exciting cause of the onset of neurotic illness lies in the external factor which may generally be described as *frustration*. The person was healthy as long as his erotic need was satisfied by an actual object in the outer world ; he becomes neurotic as soon as he is deprived of this object and no substitute is forthcoming. Happiness here coincides with health, unhappiness with neurosis. By providing a substitute for the lost source of gratification, fate can effect a cure more easily than the physician."[1]

" . . . There are only two ways possible of retaining

[1] Sigmund Freud. *A General Selection Psycho-Analytical Epitomes,* pages 7of.

health in a continuous state of frustration of satisfaction : first, that of transposing the mental tension into active energy which remains directed towards the outer world and finally wrests from that world an actual satisfaction for the libido ; and secondly, that of renouncing the libidinal satisfaction, subliminating the stored up libido and making use of it to ends which are no longer erotic and thus elude the frustration. Both possibilities can be realized in the destinies of mankind, which shows that unhappiness does not necessarily coincide with neurosis, and frustration not alone decisive for the health or ill-health of the person concerned."[1]

What happens when libido is frustrated ? The frustrated impulses then follow a psychological law and resort to phantasy. The law is : Any impulse unsatisfied in reality tends to create its object in phantasy. The frustrated energy may regress and in that case the content of the phantasy will come from re-animated experiences of childhood. These memories would come into the mind with a sort of attraction as though we desired to repeat these experiences. In phantasy we re-live these erotic experiences and embellish them by our later knowledge. These phantasies are contrary to our adult ideals and cultural leanings. Hence a conflict results between the tendency to phantasy and the ego which is still accessible to the cultural standards. The individual may then attempt to repress the conflicting tendencies and symptoms begin to appear, and may end in neurotic illness. This is why Freud argues that the symptoms represent substitute gratifications. The conclusion to which Freud comes is : " That the whole process originates in the actual frustration."

If the individual attempts to seize a gratification inconsistent with the cultural ideals of the individual, that attempt is met by the super-ego or, as I call it, the prohibitive conscience within the individual's own mind. In other words, the

[1] Ibid., page 71.

9

individual is confronted by the inner voice which demands moral control and submission to the prohibitions of conscience. If the prohibition is strong enough to overcome the attempt to seize the gratification without modifying the individual's desire, repression begins and symptom formation takes place.

In both cases the individual falls ill because *he could not adapt to the frustration.*

Now, the point I want to make is that even if we grant Freud's position (and there can be no question but that frustration often does lie at the origins of illness), it is not the deprivation of the erotic need that is the causative factor, *but the incapacity to deal with it.* As we have seen, Freud admits that frustration is not alone decisive for the health or ill-health of the person concerned. The deprivation is the occasion of the illness, not the cause. The cause lies in defective character-structure. A mature character has the capacity to endure tension, either moral or appetitive. Freud implies this when he complains that many of his patients refused or found it hard to renounce immediate pleasures for others which, even if they are longer delayed, are still real.[1]

Hence, when we speak of a man suffering from sex repression it should be understood that it is not sex which is the vital factor but the repression of it. Repression is a form of control ; control is an expression of character. Repression is a form of control by fear and escape. The fear blocks the tendency before it enters awareness ; it then causes a " flight into psychological disease ". Thus repression is a personality-disorder because the manner in which we control our behaviour-tendencies is a character trait. Our mental and spiritual health do not depend on our behaviour-tendencies but on the manner in which we control them ; and that is fundamentally a matter of character.

There are people who do not resort to repression ; they

[1] Ibid., page 112.

may have perverted behaviour-tendencies and yet they do not fall ill, or manifest distressing symptoms. Some even glory in their perversions and attempt to justify them. Others accept the perverted tendencies and face and control them in consciousness. Consequently there is no nervous breakdown. It is an axiom of psychotherapy that tendencies which are conscious, conflicts which are not repressed, may cause much spiritual distress and temptation, but they cannot create a nervous symptom, at least of the more distressing type. It is not sex, then, which is the constant factor in neurotic trouble but repression. As we shall see later, the character trait which is expressed in the fact of repression is itself repressed. Repression[1] is really the refusal of the self to integrate impulses or tendencies into the organized personality. Hence we can conclude that before repression has been resorted to integration has failed from one reason or another. Repression, however, we shall study later. Meantime, we are just concerned to show that it is not instinctual drives which lie at the root of either neurotic trouble or character-disturbance, but the repression of them ; and that repression is due to a character-structure.

Progress in the understanding of neurotic trouble and personality disorders can only come as we widen our concept of causative factors. No psychotherapist will deny that in the majority of people he sees sex difficulties come to the surface sooner or later. In some the whole difficulty is that of dealing rightly with sex. Both Adler and Jung, who broke with the Freudian theory of sex, admit the prevalence of sex conflict ; and Karen Horney, in her *New Ways of Psychoanalysis*, does not attempt to deny how prominent a feature sex difficulties are. But these difficulties are, in a great many individuals, secondary and not primary. As we said before,

[1] Cf. Stekel. *Conditions of Nervous Anxiety and Their Treatment*, page 6.

sex difficulties may be cleared up, yet the basic anxiety still remain. There are also many cases in which we do not find any sex difficulties at all. So far as my own experience goes, I found that when I dealt with the character of the patient rather than with his childhood experiences of sex ; or when I dealt with the reactions to an early sex experience rather than concentrate on the experience itself, I made far more rapid progress. Otherwise I found I simply alleviated the symptoms and did not cure. I also found that concentrating thus on the character-structure of the patient the sex difficulties cleared up with the patient's efforts to correct his character-formations. It seems to me that a truer psychopathology of all these disturbances will be found when we realize that complexes are the result of character-formations and not character-formations the outcome of complexes.

We are now in a position to appreciate the contributions being made to personality-psychology by such thinkers as Erich Fromm[1] and Karen Horney.[2] The latter speaks of Neurotic Needs and not of complexes, such as *the neurotic need for affection*. These neurotic needs are not mere complexes ; they are not besetting sins on which we have to keep a watchful eye ; they are not the outcome of a behaviour tendency which has had to be dissociated and makes its presence known by a particular phobia or definite hysterical symptoms, or in a particular anxiety situation. They are trends which belong to character-structure. These character-trends determine the reaction to what Karen Horney calls " basic anxiety ".

Perhaps our later discussion will be clearer if we get a thorough understanding of this concept. There is a type of neurosis which, as a rule, clears up rather quickly. Those

---

[1] *The Fear of Freedom.*

[2] *The Neurotic Personality of Our Time. New Ways in Psycho-Analysis. Self-Analysis.*

who fall into it are not of the neurotic type at all. They have come up against a situation in which they repress an element of a conflict which the situation has created. I had a woman sent to me who, from all appearances, seemed to be a very sensible and balanced individual. Inwardly she was full of anxiety, and had been afraid of hurting her child. She had been treated for glandular disease for six months without the anxiety being allayed. When the trouble was exposed it was not difficult to clear the whole thing up. She had one child and she and her husband had discussed the idea of having another. There was the difficulty of the war ; her husband was of military age although reserved for the time being. Through one difficulty or another the discussion went on for twelve months. Finally they decided to have a baby and almost immediately the woman suffered terrors of anxiety. During her first pregnancy she had not been well at all ; and the birth was a long and difficult one. Consciously she did not seem to mind having a baby, or rather she was keen to have one. Something in the unconscious resisted the idea strenuously. She had submitted to the idea and her submission had created hostile feelings against the idea of having a baby ; these hostile feelings were displaced upon the child she already had. There was hostility against her husband. When they had discussed the baby, little or nothing had been said about the possibility of another bad time. *That was repressed.* The whole situation was analysed out, and the symptoms steadily disappeared until they cleared up entirely. By the time they cleared up the woman had taken a perfectly spontaneous attitude to another baby.

The neurosis here was entirely due to a situation which had not been squarely faced. No character-change was needed. Normally the woman had no more anxiety than the ordinary housewife with a growing child.

Where there is " basic anxiety ", or " basic hostility ",

however, we have a very different situation, and one that does not clear up quickly. At the root of every character-neurosis there is basic anxiety and probably also basic hostility. It arises in the attitude a child takes to the world. It may originate in some experience in childhood in which the child has been made to feel a deep sense of guilt and fear ; or in some situation in which the child has lost the sense of security. This sense of insecurity or fear of doing wrong becomes a part of the child's psychic make-up or, in the terms we have been using, a character-structure. It determines the attitude of the growing child not to one situation but to every situation ; so that when adulthood is reached even ordinary happenings which, to a normal person, would cause no more than a little worry or anxiety stimulate intense anxiety.

A good example of this basic anxiety is seen in another woman who for years has suffered intense melancholic feelings at the thought of what people must suffer if they have done some wrong. She feels as guilty as if she had herself done the thing. The very mention of the word " sin " or " forgiveness " can make her feel intensely unhappy. Her mind is continually working to be reassured that God is love, that we have just to be sorry for anything we have done wrong to be restored to a relationship of harmony with God. Her psychological attitude was well brought out in a dream. She dreamed she was taken before the Spanish Inquisition. When she looked at them gathered round a table at once the thought came to her mind : " I must keep on the right side of these people." There you have her whole psychology as far as religion is concerned. God is one that you must keep on the right side of. That created a perfectionist trend in her character-structure. She must do nothing wrong ; temptation must not assail her ; sexual sins especially must be avoided. Responsibility for marital relations must rest on the husband. There were found in the analysis the usual incidents of sexual play characteristic of children ; and the memory of them carried a great amount of guilt-feeling. Her anxiety about people suffering continuous guilt-feelings for anything they had done wrong was mostly connected with those who had illegitimate children, or were pregnant before marriage. Her sex relations with her husband were normal. The Freudians would put everything down to the sex repression. This, however, is to fail to understand the condition. Her sex impulses could not be integrated with her personality while she held this attitude to God as one Who snoops around for sinners. With those impulses un-integrated she must feel a sense of insecurity. The whole thing dated back to an after-prayer meeting in her church. What was said by the speaker or in the prayers we have never been able to get back ; perhaps it was a general feeling or attitude she introjected. Whatever it was, the result was that the formation of a character-neurosis which compelled her to experience a sense of insecurity and guilt-feelings against which she had to defend herself by projecting the guilt-feelings into others' minds ; and to protect herself from any such sins she develops the perfectionist trend which compelled her to avoid " sin ", and yet to flog herself for supposed flaws within herself.

Such a neurosis cannot be cleared up in a few interviews. The whole attitude to religion and to life must be altered. In her unconscious mind she must cling to this wrong idea of God ; she needs it to protect herself against any wrong-doing. She has submitted, as Erich Fromm would say, to this idea of God ; and the submission has generated a rebellious drive against it. The prohibitive conscience or " super-ego " whose ideational content is this threatening God blocks everything but the guilt-feelings. No wonder she says that every day is an agony.

It would not be untrue to say that every neurotic is a human being suffering from a sense of insecurity, and that the character-structure has been formed with a view to defending the individual against anxiety which a sense of insecurity can generate. When we remember that the Behaviourists have shown that the sense of insecurity is one of the conditions of arousing innate fear we get confirmation from a quarter that is apt to be neglected.

How dangerous it is, however, to make generalizations attempting to embrace the whole field can be seen when we have to tell of character-structures which are designed to allow the prohibited tendencies to get gratification without guilt. Yet the two explanations are not so far apart as one might imagine. The fact that the individual has to take " surreptitious " ways in getting gratifications of his behaviour-tendencies shows that he is really afraid of guilt-feelings, and feels insecure against the disapproval of others.

We must note here that with the sense of insecurity there is always associated hostile feelings which may express them-selves in violent tempers and even in acts of violence. More often than not they are repressed ; with the result that the individual feels more insecure tha ι ever. These hostile feelings, as Erich Fromm has pointe l out in relation to the child who has submitted to the pare ts, are directed against the very persons on whom the indi idual depends for his security. If it is the world in ge ieral that makes the individual feel insecure, then the hosti ty will be felt against the world as such. If it is one's religic ιs beliefs that is at the root of the hostility there will be hostile feelings against God. One woman had such hostility against God that she had a compulsive tendency to offer her prayers to the Devil, or to give her soul to the Devil as though she could spite God.

A good example is seen in a rather brilliant young man who was is a good position. His immediate superior he felt " picked his brains ". He had no degree, and in the race for promotion the man with a degree generally won. This increased his hostility. He repressed the hostility ; became apprehensive and sometimes depressed. He felt on occasions a rush of feeling which invariably made him almost sick with feelings of panic. The root of the trouble was that subconsciously he felt that at any moment he would lose control of his feelings, or say something which no self-respecting superior could pass over, and he would thus lose his job.

In the last lecture, when we come to deal with the origin and nature of conflict, we shall hear more about these character-neuroses, or rather the character-trends which give rise to these. Enough has now been said to show that he who would understand the conflicts of the human soul must understand a great deal more than the catalogue of instincts given by McDougall, or the complexes mentioned by Freud. Freud explains life as though it were a continual striving against instinctual drives ; McDougall does lay stress on the sentiments within which the instincts become organized and sees in the integration of these sentiments the character of the individual. But even he did not believe that there were any ends outside instinctive drives, or propensities, as he came later to call them. Both McDougall and Freud proceed as though man, or rather human nature, was a fixed condition, and as though human nature was to be found in the physiological drives alone. It is true that we have drives which determine that we shall defend ourselves against danger, that we shall eat, sleep and reproduce our kind. There is nothing fixed about these drives, however. They can reach a state of tension through lack of satisfaction which becomes unbearable, especially those connected with the need for self-preservation. It is a mistake to conclude from these primary needs that the form of satisfaction is fixed. They are really physiological drives and not instincts. Perhaps it would be more accurate if we dropped using the term " instinct " in regard to man altogether. Man has certain fundamental needs connected with the organism such as the need for self-preservation ; and certain needs connected with the development of personality ; he has a need to run his life by some kind of standard of values ; he has a need for a meaning to life ; he has a need to be recognized as a person. In other words, he has needs which pertain to his organic being and needs which pertain to his spiritual being. We are unlikely to understand man unless we realize that he is the creature of a two dimensional world—a temporal and a spiritual. These needs he neglects at his peril. That these needs may be frustrated is common ground to all schools of psychological thought. Neurotic illness, however, is not caused by the frustration but is due to the reactions we take to the frustrated needs. The frustration in itself could not cause neurotic trouble ; and the notion that all neurotic trouble is the outcome of frustrated sexual libido has to be abandoned. No doubt we find that many victims of neurotic diseases have sexual troubles ; but so have people who show no signs of neurotic troubles.

The root of the troubles must be looked for in the kind of adaptation the individual has made to life in general and to the social situation he finds himself in particular. Biological needs must be integrated with personality needs ; pleasures must be integrated with moral values ; the demands of adulthood call for a steady transference of interests which were perfectly legitimate in childhood or adolescence to the interests consistent with the responsibilities of a grown-up. Some kind of adjustment has to be made to social reality ; social reality is never static ; it is for ever exerting an influence on us in the sense already explained, namely that we must somehow fit into it or change it if it has become too rigid for individuals to reach the " prospective aim of personality ". We begin our mental career with minds whose content is derived from the social process. Hence the social and cultural situation in which we grow up is not external to us ; we internalize social values, social attitudes and social prohibitions. These are emotionally rooted before we even know the meaning of the terms. They are not concepts which we may change without alteration of our character ; they are our character and can only be changed by changing something of our outlook on life, and the structure of our inner being.

Neurotic trouble then is the outcome of inner conflict ; it is a conflict between these internalized values, attitudes and prohibitions and the drive of organic or personality needs. We may call all these drives of our organisms and personality " wants " with T. H. Green. The mere satisfying of these wants will not satisfy man. Man's satisfactions lie in what Green called " wanted objects ". This is to say, one cannot divorce the satisfaction of wants from the kind of objects through which we satisfy the wants. I may seek a " wanted object " that may be forbidden by society. I have then to adjust myself to the prohibition ; I have to adapt myself to the approvals of society and my character is formed through such adaptations. If I fail to adjust myself and satisfy the want then the drive that belongs to personality as a whole, what we have called " the prospective aim of personality ", may be thwarted, and a conflict begins within myself. On the other hand, I may feel that the prohibitions or conventions of society are curbing the natural freedom without which the prospective aim of personality cannot be reached. That will be a perfectly conscious state of mind ; it may lead to a conscious attempt to alter social values or standards. Such a conflict may be exhilarating and is not at all neurotic ; it is the fight for freedom ; it is the warfare from which says the Scripture there is no discharge.

The kind of adjustment we make to social process becomes

part of our character-structure, a habitual mode of reaction, whether that reaction is by feeling, conation or idea. On that character-structure depends our mental and spiritual health ; it is that which must be changed when we fall ill of a neurosis, or find debilitating spiritual conflicts within ourselves that hinder our spiritual life.

In closing this chapter it is well to remind ourselves that not all disturbances in the realm of character, nor those illnesses which manifest themselves in psychological symptoms, can be laid at the door of mental causes. The youthful science of Endocrinology shows conclusively that certain nervous symptoms as well as certain disturbances of character may be due to glandular disease. Diseases of the thyroid gland are always accompanied by emotional changes in the sufferer ; and there are strong grounds for believing that disturbances of the pituitary gland and delinquency are intimately connected.[1] There are grounds, also, for believing that emotional and mental disturbance can effect the glandular balance and thus accentuate the symptoms. What is cause and what is effect here seem difficult to estimate. Not seldom a patient is treated for glandular disturbance but the symptoms do not yield to the treatment. The same patient may respond almost at once to psychotherapy. Dr. Harrow, in his *Glands in Health and Disease*,[2] says : "It may not be amiss to point out that the psychic factor in the treatment of hyperthyroidism cannot be overlooked. Psycho-analysis, handled by pseudo-scientists, has become a laughing stock, just as the glandular treatment and the general subject of ductless glands threatens to become ; but psychotherapy practised by the skilful physician is at times of inestimable aid in putting the patient on his feet."

[1] See *An Introduction to Psychological Medicine*, by Fraser, Harris and Rees, page 197.
[2] Page 35.

There are, however, too many unsolved problems in the field of glandular therapy for any enthusiast in this branch of medicine to speak of " a chemistry of the soul " ; and just as the administration of drugs can alleviate definite psychological conditions, so it would seem that the application of psychological principles can help to alleviate the emotional upset caused by a disturbance of the glandular balance.

The after-effects of " sleepy-sickness " has peculiar manifestations on some of the victims of this disease. Some may suffer real physical impairment which leaves behind symptoms such as a severe tremor, and a lack of co-ordinated movement ; others may suffer apparently little or no physical impairment as far as movement is concerned, but their character undergoes a change. Whereas there was no previous sign of delinquency in the individual before the illness, the patient has now to fight or yields to criminal tendencies.

Nor must we forget that diseases of the central nervous system have their psychological effects. No psychological treatment can be of any use where there is deterioration of the nerve cells.

Hence we must not assume that every psychological effect is due to a psychological cause. There is no sphere in which we should remember more the logical doctrine of " Plurality of causes " as in medicine.

Apart from physical disease there are diseases of psychological origin which are altogether outside the sphere of pastoral psychology. There is a clear distinction between the psycho-neuroses and the psychoses. " The psychoses include those conditions which have been popularly covered by the word ' insanity '. They are mental disorders in which emotional, intellectual and volitional upset is so great that the ability of the individual to adapt himself to life as a whole is seriously affected. The person suffering from one of these disorders becomes a danger to himself or a disturbing influence on the life of the community."[1] The Manic-depressive psychoses, Involutional Melancholia, the Schizophrenic reaction types and Paranoia, should be left entirely alone so far as Pastoral Psychology is concerned. Institutional treatment should always be recommended. In the psychoneuroses such as Neurasthenia, Anxiety-states, the Obsession-Compulsion states, the patients as a rule are perfectly conscious that the trouble is within themselves, although they are unconscious as to why they should have the symptoms ; and also they have good insight. These two conditions are necessary for all psychotherapeutic treatment.

Later in the course we shall see how far the pastor and medical practitioner can co-operate in those disturbances, which are ultimately due to character-structure. That there is a wide field for co-operation no one who knows the subject will deny. Last winter I lectured to a society composed of doctors, clergy 'and social workers in Derby, whose main object is to see how far doctors and clergy can co-operate, and the two recognized psychiatrists who were present at practically every lecture showed a keen interest in the character-aspect of these nervous diseases with which they deal every day. But co-operation must depend on the pastor having a clear knowledge of the limitations of psychology as well as of a knowledge of psychological processes. If the temptation of the ordinary practitioner is to become irritable with his neurotic patients, the danger of many pastors is to over-simplify the causes of the trouble ; and thus he attempts to deal with individuals who need specialist's treatment.

[1] *An Introduction to Psychological Medicine,* by Fraser, etc., Chapter I.

PSYCHOLOGY, PSYCHOTHERAPY AND PASTORAL PSYCHOLOGY

It will be well, at this point, to define some of the terms and to get a clear understanding of some of the most important mental processes studied in psychological medicine, and to see what their application is to Pastoral Psychology.

Psychology itself we may define as the science of the mental processes which manifest themselves in ideas, emotions and behaviour-tendencies, and of the processes whereby we arrive at our knowledge of the external world. The second part of the definition covers what is known as the older metaphysical psychology. We may compress the definition and say: Psychology is the science of the mental processes whereby the self becomes aware of itself, and whereby it knows, feels and behaves.

A good deal of modern psychology ignores the self or subject whose processes it studies. Mental processes, however, are always the experiences of a subject that is capable of knowing the processes experienced, and indeed capable of modifying those processes. The self is conscious of itself as subject; it is not merely an object like a piece of matter; it has initiative, the capacity for self-direction and self-control. Matter behaves; but as far as we know the behaviour is not an experience. We can study the processes involved in suffering, but suffering is essentially an experience of a self; there are cognitive processes; but knowing or cognition is essentially an experience of a subject who knows what it is experiencing. When we modify mental processes we modify the self; and the self can take a hand in changing or modifying the processes. The study of self-hood, in our opinion, is

23

an essential part of the science of psychology. If, as we have contended, neuroticism or personality-disorder is the outcome of character-structure, then it follows that it is the self which is defective and not merely a mental process; for character, as James Ward taught us, can be predicated only of a self. When we speak of a dissociated self we mean a self that has lost its " togetherness "—one of the main marks of self-hood. There is no anxiety-state apart from a self that is anxious and apprehensive. It is the self we must change and not a mere process. I remember a patient who, when she came with a dream that was not very complimentary to her, used to say: " Oh, that is the patient's dream, not mine." Not until she was willing to realize that her dreams were an expression of herself could she make progress. Until the self takes a hand in changing its ways of behaving, feeling and thinking, the psychotherapist or pastor is helpless.

Psychotherapy is the application of psychological principles to the treatment of disorders whose origin lies in mental factors; that is to say, whose origin lies in the ideas, emotions or impulses of the self. It is not a science but an art. Nevertheless, from the observation of what happens when psychological principles are applied it may come to add· to our knowledge of psychological fact.

Psychopathology, on the other hand, is a science. As Dr. Bernhard Hart puts it: " Psychopathology connotes, not a mere description of mental symptoms, but an endeavour to explain disorder or certain disorders in terms of psychological processes."[1] In other words, psychopathology cannot be satisfied with a mere description of mental symptoms; description of mental symptoms is the task of clinical psychiatry; and not until the student studies the mental processes which are the causative factors of the symptoms, does he reach the science of psychopathology.

[1] Bernhard Hart. *Psychopathology*, page 8.

Psychiatry is often equated with psychotherapy. If there is any distinction of meaning it is found in the fact that the psychotherapist confines himself to the treatment of the psychoneuroses, whereas the psychiatrist also treats the true insanities, or the psychoses.

Now, in what sense can we use the term Pastoral Psychology ? Is it a science like psychology and psychopathology ? Or is it an art like psychiatry and psychotherapy ? Actually it is both a science and an art. Like psychotherapy and psychopathology, it is dependent on psychology for its knowledge of psychological principles. It shares the psychotherapist's interest in the removal of symptoms ; but it goes further ; it is much more concerned with the unification of the self. Like the psychopathologist, it seeks for the causes of the trouble and believes that ultimately the causes of personality-disturbances are to be found in a wrong relation to spiritual things, or, in other words, to God. Its field is wider than that of either psychotherapy or psychopathology. These are mostly concerned with the mental processes which incapacitate the individual and make him maladjusted to life. Pastoral Psychology, on the other hand, has for its field the understanding of the development of character in normal people, and especially it studies the relation of religious beliefs to the development of character and its stability, and to the achievement of personality. Disturbances of character and the sense of guilt it explains in terms of ethics and theology. Although it calls envy, pride, wrath and lust sins, it does not deny that these sins can become pathological and that they can become accentuated through the process of repression, and consequently should be treated by the psychotherapist. It would contend with Jung, however, that these pathological trends of character cannot be really cured unless the patient comes consciously under the influence of religious ideals. It emphasizes the fact that the mere bringing of the repressed tendency into consciousness does not of itself cure ; the patient, if he is to be rid of the tendency or is to bring it under conscious control, must make a moral decision regarding it ; he must get spiritual insight into the meaning of his symptoms or behaviour-tendencies.

Here is a patient, for example, suffering from anxiety and apprehensiveness. The root of the trouble is a repressed promiscuous tendency. He is now made conscious of the tendency ; he is conscious also that he repressed it lest the temptation to adultery should have been too strong for him to overcome ; he is now aware of the temptation. He has now to make a decision about it.

Here is a woman with what Karen Horney calls *the Neurotic Need for a Partner.*[1] She is afraid to stay in the house alone or to go out alone. Her love is parasitic and she has a compulsive need for the husband's affection. Her love is purely ego-centric and she will give love to anyone of either sex who seems to her to offer this affection she is compulsively seeking. She has marked hysterical symptoms. She is wholly concerned with his feelings towards her, not her own feelings towards her husband. Along with her " affection " she has violent feelings towards him. She feels insecure against the world and against her own impulses. He must be her protector ; he must be there just when she wants him ; he must come up to all her expectations of him ; otherwise the violent feelings are let loose. All this she becomes conscious of during analysis. But if she is to be cured she has to see herself in a moral perspective, and she has to do something about it. Unless she comes to a decision about it, she will be in the same dangers from which her symptoms were a psychological escape.

From these two examples we can see that Pastoral

[1] *Self-Analysis*, page 55.

Psychology comes in after the psychotherapist has done his work. Patients have not only to be saved from their repressions and sense of guilt but they have to be made safe. Pastoral Psychology completes the work of psychotherapy.

Pastoral Psychology differs in its function from psychotherapy, or rather, it has a function which psychotherapy does not claim to perform. The psychotherapist does not as a rule see people unless they are driven to him by a sense of inadequacy ; their condition has become pathological before they call in his help. Pastoral Psychology has a preventive function. In the hands of a true spiritual director it can prevent repression and hence neurotic trouble.

One application of this is seen in the Roman Catholic Confessional. It cannot be a mere coincidence that psychotherapists see very few Roman Catholics. Dr. Jung tells us that in his international practice he has not seen more than half a dozen people who belong to that religious persuasion. In over twenty years' practice I have treated not more than that number. Two of these were married to protestants and one was a professional man who had turned in his thirties to that religion.

Two reasons I think can be given for this influence of the Confessional and the spiritual direction given by the Roman Catholic Church. In the first place, although Roman Catholicism is severe in its condemnation of sinful tendencies, it lays the emphasis upon the mercy of God and His willingness to forgive sin. It stresses on the mind of the penitent the frailty of the flesh. The priest who is strictly trained in moral theology knows how to calm the fears, alleviate the sense of guilt, and deal with the moral scruples of the distressed soul. Very, very often I have quoted to someone heavily burdened by a sense of guilt a passage from Father Grou's *Manual for Interior Souls*, which has helped, for the time being at least, to lift the burden. The passage is worth quoting as an example of the kind of spiritual direction which can prevent repression as well as help to lift it. " The truly devout man ", he writes, " has a determination, once and for all, to refuse nothing to God, to grant nothing to self-love, and never to commit a voluntary fault ; but he does not perplex himself ; he goes on courageously ; he is not over-scrupulous. If he falls into a fault, he does not agitate himself ; he humbles himself at the sight of his weakness ; he raises himself up and thinks no more about it.

" He is not astonished at his weakness, at his falls or his imperfections ; he is never discouraged. He knows that he can do nothing, but that God can do everything. He does not rely upon his own good thoughts and resolutions, but simply upon the grace and goodness of God. If he were to fall a hundred times a day he would not despair, but would stretch out his hands lovingly to God, and beg of Him to lift him up and to take pity on him.

" The truly devout man has a horror of evil, but he has a still greater love of good. He thinks more of practising virtue than about avoiding vice."[1]

This is an example of true spiritual direction. It has real psychological insight, and shows the way in which one should treat the sense of guilt and weakness, whether the individual is conscious or unconscious of the source of guilt and temptation. Practically every sufferer from guilt of a morbid kind is more afraid of evil than he is in love with the good ; and is very apt to spend all his moral strength not in trying to be good, but in trying not to be bad.

Such people suffer from what the psycho-analyst calls " a ruthless super ego " ; or, as I should express it, from a severe prohibitive conscience which they have failed to outgrow. A great deal of pastoral direction should aim at

---

[1] Quoted in *The Way to God*, edited by Sir James Marchant, K.B.E., pp. 10, 11 (published by Burns, Oates and Washbourne).

lessening the intolerance of this prohibitive conscience. It is not easy for those who have compulsive tendencies to evil to realize that their faults are compulsive ; they feel that they are coerced, and yet they flog themselves unmercifully. If the spiritual director can reduce the intolerance of the prohibitive conscience he gives the individual the chance to see that he is the victim of a compulsive tendency that must be altered and can only be altered by a change of character.

The second reason for the good psychological effects of the Roman Confessional lies in the fact that the handling of guilt such as that expressed in the quotation prevents the Catholic from repressing the tendency or character-structure into the unconscious ; and consequently the individual is kept from neuroticism and encouraged to acknowledge his weakness and to rely upon God. At the same time he is re-enforced in his attempt to repudiate the tendencies, and to bring them under self-control. It is a truism of psychotherapy that behaviour-tendencies which are conscious cannot create a neurotic symptom. They may cause moral and spiritual distress ; they can make temptation hard to withstand, but as long as the conflict remains within consciousness no debilitating symptom can be formed.

Hence the wise spiritual director never humiliates his penitents nor loses patience with them ; he knows that humiliation makes a man look down on himself, whereas true humility makes the individual look up to God. When the Roman Catholic receives absolution the sins are buried. We Protestants, on the other hand, have the bad habit, as Dr. Maltby once said, of giving them a prolonged funeral. There is nothing like a prolonged funeral of our sins to bring them to life again. When the sinner is assured of absolution there is an end of it ; he is encouraged to think no more about it, and to be up and doing. That was the position of of the late Professor James : repentance, he argued, was not a grovelling over sins committed but a rising and shaking oneself free from the guilt-feelings and turning to that which is good. The Catholic priest, well trained in moral theology, is not satisfied with reassurance, although he knows the value of that in those with tendencies to morbid guilt-feelings; he helps his parishioners to be better prepared to meet the subtleties of the offending behaviour-tendencies.

Explain it as we will, there can be no question from the psychological point of view of the healthy effect of the Confessional. It is difficult for the psychologist to believe in the evils of the Confessional when he has so much evidence of its power to prevent mental and moral disturbance. One thing is certain: the fact that confession tends to keep the behaviour-tendencies in consciousness gives the opportunity to bring them under self-control and, after all, that is the solution of moral problems.

Before I leave the Confessional and its good effects, there is one curious phenomenon to note. Many members of the Catholic persuasion of the Anglican Church go regularly to Confession; but we cannot say that we have a lesser number of members of the Anglo-Catholic body as patients than of some of the Protestant Churches. Indeed, I must confess that some of the worst sufferers from morbid guilt I have seen were practising members of Anglo-Catholicism and went regularly to Confession until Confession became a nightmare. I am unable to explain this fact; and must be content merely to state it.

The wider function of Pastoral Psychology is again seen in the fact that the pastor, as preacher as well as priest, has for his primary function the task of giving to his people a religious meaning to life. Already we have seen that Dr. Jung's position is that " A psychoneurosis must be understood as the suffering of a human being who has not discovered what life means for him." In other words, to remain mentally healthy the individual needs a philosophy of life. The theologian would probably put it that the individual must be reconciled to God. But that is just the same thing in religious terms ; for to know what life means for me is to have a philosophy of life and it is to have come to terms with God.

That this philosophy of life is needed can be easily understood when we realize that all neurotic trouble and personality-disturbance is due ultimately to a sense of insecurity which may or may not be conscious. The character-structure of the neurotic is formed in the attempts to defend himself against this sense of insecurity. That we shall see when we come to the study of the nature and origin of conflict.

Meantime, it is being more and more recognized by psychotherapists that a philosophy of life is a foundation of the stable and healthy mental life. In their *Introduction to Psychological Medicine*, the writers, in their chapter dealing with Personality, say that a man's philosophy of life "is his guiding principle, according to which he models his actions and arranges his ideas. . . .

"The philosophy of life may be and frequently is a religion, but it is not necessarily so ; hence it is better to use the more general term. This must obviously be closely associated with the sentiment of self-regard, for without a reasonably defined philosophy of life there can be no clear conception in the individual's own mind of what his relationships are to his environment. It has been said that the trouble with the psychoneurotic is that he has lost or never developed a philosophy of life with the result he is like a rudderless ship on an uncharted sea. There is a good deal of truth in this, and the organization of the sentiment of self-regard with an adequate philosophy of life constitutes the final mental organization.

"As a result of this organization and implicit in it, there

emerges what is called Will, which is the final conative product. Will is the impulse to action organized at fully conscious levels."[1] That means that a philosophy of life not only gives direction to our behaviour-tendencies but gives a goal to the Will.

This is a more cautious statement than that of Dr. Jung. Nevertheless it confirms our contention about the relation of a philosophy of life to mental health and the stability of the personality.

Now, Pastoral Psychology alone has the right to enter this field. Freud and the analytical school repudiate the idea that it is any of their business to give a man a philosophy of life ; the psychotherapist does not admit that he is required to have a finished outlook on life, and his professional conscience does not demand it of him. But the primary task of the pastor, priest or preacher is just to do this very thing. Thus it would seem that Pastoral Psychology, from the point of view of mental health and the achievement of personality, is the more important discipline than either psychopathology or psychotherapy. Dr. Ranyard West, in a recent volume on *Conscience and Society*, seems to think that most mental illnesses are rooted in misconceptions. There is a very great deal of truth in his contention : misconceptions regarding God, of ethical demands, and of human nature undoubtedly play a large part in neurotic trouble. Misconceptions often lie beneath the sense of insecurity against which the neurotic is unconsciously defending himself. It would be a mistake, however, to think that therapy consists in removing intellectual misconceptions. That would be an over-simplification indeed.

Now, a philosophy of life in the academic sense very few people have ; it is, for the great majority of people, contained in their religious faith and beliefs. Often that philosophy is contained in the simplest of hymns, but a life organized round

[1] Page 55.

the ideas cannot but be stable. Over the wireless came the other Sunday evening a service from the Salvation Army. I forget all the rest of the service, but a verse of a hymn which I had not heard before. Here it is, as far as I can remember it :

> " All your anxiety and all your care,
>   Bring to the Mercy-seat and leave it there.
>   There is never a burden he cannot share ;
>   There is no friend like Jesus."

The philosopher or psychologist in us might be inclined to sneer at such a " Come to Jesus " theology ; but is the meaning very different from the passage of the late Professor James : " How can it possibly fail to cool the fever, appease the fret and steady the nerves, if one is sensibly conscious of the fact that one is in the keeping of One whom we can absolutely trust ? "[1]

Certainly it is not for the psychologist or psychotherapist to be concerned that his patient should have a certain philosophy or a definite type of religion. He cannot, however, leave religious questions alone ; there are few patients who do not relate their troubles to religious difficulties of one kind or another. The pastor's task is to give an adequate meaning to life ; and its adequacy must be measured by the power it gives to the individual to meet the difficulties of life without escaping into neurosis. The importance of conveying this meaning to life, or conveying religion in a healthy form is supreme.

There is another branch of Pastoral Psychology which is just as important as that of conveying to each generation a healthy form of religion. It has the task of building up the interior life of the soul, both in its relation to God and to men. This branch of Pastoral Psychology has a long tradition

[1] *Varities of Religious Experience.*

behind it. It was taught under the heading of Moral and Ascetic Theology. Many of its teachers had a very fine capacity for introspection and a wonderful power of describing mental states. Dr. McCurdy says that the description of depression by John of Damascus could not be bettered ;[1] while Bishop Paget paraphrases an excellent description of Acedia by St. Thomas Aquinas.

Unfortunately, we Non-conformists have shown little capacity here ; and indeed not very much interest ; so that we are the worst equipped to deal with the interior difficulties of our people. We have no spiritual technique. Our Summer Schools and " Retreat " days can give an intellectual stimulus and provide healthy contact with other ministers ; but one could not say that they are designed to unify the interior life of the soul. The technique of Evangelical Conventions, such as that of the famous Keswick Convention, is a good technique for the mass production of spiritual emotionalism ; and I doubt not has a good effect in many ways ; and as a by-product it may inspire many a man or woman to find a spiritual technique for themselves. " The quiet time " of the Oxford Group has many dangers. To be able to listen to God is the fruit of a well-disciplined soul and scarcely a technique for beginners. Unless the soul is well-disciplined " wishful thinking " will be mistaken for the voice of God ; and many of the directions I have heard groupers recount as received in their " quiet time " seemed to me to be simple inferences which ought to need no special technique at all. The very fact, however, that such a technique was felt to be necessary and was developed shows that non-sacramentarian religion felt the need of it.

The cultivation of the spiritual life has been subordinate to the development of the intellectual side of our religious experience. This is certainly a mistake, as both sides of our

[1] *The Psychology of Emotion*, page 343.

spiritual life should not only walk in step ; but both sides should bear each other's burdens. In Professor H. G. Paton's *The Good Will* he argues that " the apprehension of goodness is not merely an intellectual matter, but demands for its possibility the presence of a particular kind of will ".[1] The same thing is true in this sphere of religious experience : the apprehension of religious truth depends for its possibility on the presence of an interior life which is spiritually developed. There is an introverted side of religious experience on which the extraverted side depends for its healthiness. We Nonconformists tend to order the spiritual life as though we were all extraverts, and forget the introverted types whose religious experience is much more inclined to be interior. Actually a true interior religious life gives balance to the extraverted types, while the objective forms of worship of the sacramentarians tend to balance and keep healthy the introverted type of religious mind.

Spiritual technique should be designed so as to provide for three fundamental needs of personality. Our behaviour-tendencies need to be organized within sentiments. When our tendencies are organized within sentiments they become subordinate to some end ; they become controlled by our personality as a whole and there is very much less danger of impulsive behaviour ; or, to put it simply, there is less danger that we shall be at the mercy of every passing desire. The sex tendencies, e.g. are never safe until they are organized within a love sentiment for one of the opposite sex. When they are so organized the pleasures of sex are fused with the joy and happiness of love ; and their exercise tends to increase the love. Our moral sentiment or conscience has for its end the regulation and co-ordination of our behaviour-tendencies in accord with whatever ideals we have consciously or unconsciously accepted. To the extent that our moral senti-

[1] Page 20.

ment is truly assimilated and thus truly our own and not merely the outcome of the authority of our teachers, our inclinations and will tend to coincide. What we ought to do becomes synonymous with what we want to do ; and to the degree that has taken place there is less division in the soul, and character becomes closely knit. Our religious sentiment will contain much if not all our philosophy of life and will give sanction to our conscience and direction to our will. It will also, however, be the medium through which we have our religious experience ; according to its strength and activity we shall have fellowship with God ; and according to the degree that sentiment permeates all our other sentiments to that degree we shall have the second need of personality satisfied, namely the sense of security. If that sense of security is firm the third need of personality is fulfilled, namely the sense of belonging ; or, to put it the other way round, we shall have no gnawing sense of aloneness and isolation.

These three needs, the unification of our personality, the sense of security, and the sense of belonging, must be ministered to by a truly well-informed spiritual technique. They are all interior needs and until they are satisfied the external world contains for the individual an incipient hostility at least ; nor does the individual feel safe in regard to his behaviour-tendencies. Every failure to become adjusted to life, to God and our fellow-men, will be found to have at its roots the sense of insecurity, a feeling of aloneness and isolation, and repressed hostile feelings. The *enjoyment of God* should be the supreme end of spiritual technique ; and it is in that enjoyment of God we feel not only saved in the Evangelical sense, but safe ; we are conscious of belonging to God, and hence are never alone ; and, to the degree we have these two, hostile feelings disappear.

It is possible to state the same thing in another way. The relationship to God and man, and to our moral ideals should be one of spontaneity. It is not our submission God wants but our spontaneous love and fellowship ; a mere submission to moral ideals transforms that which ought to be the outcome of a free and spontaneous choice into a compulsion, and no man is safe whose morality is a compulsion. "Henceforth, I call you not servants but friends " ; that is the relationship between God and man which spiritual technique should make its supreme end to cultivate. "If you love Me you will keep my commandments " ; Christian morality springs out of this spontaneous love relationship between God and man. In that relationship Nature seems friendly and homely ; even its vast spaces instead of eliciting a sense of terror speak of the infinite love ; and the nearer beauty becomes the garment with which the Almighty clothes Himself.

It is not possible to over-emphasize this need for a simple spiritual technique which will give the religious devotee what older theologians called "assurance". A technique which will keep the soul in continuous touch with God, create in him a spontaneous love to God and the moral demands of his religion and the faith of the eighth Chapter of Romans that nothing can separate him from the love of God, is the need of every soul. Probably no one but the psychotherapist knows how widespread is this sense of insecurity and aloneness and anxiety. People do not, as a rule, speak of these things. There are many in our Churches who never feel God near, who believe in His love and yet who cannot truly say that they have experienced it ; men and women who feel intensely this aloneness and insecurity. It is on this psychological fact that we plead for a new emphasis on spiritual technique designed to give to the disciple the reality of an integrated personality, integrated by the religious sentiment —"Unite my heart to fear Thy name"—integrated in its moral ideals, and in a spontaneous relationship to Nature and man. The integration of the personality is not the act of a moment; a religious conversion may be the beginning of it, but cannot complete it; it demands spiritual discipline. McDougall argued that the closely knit character could only be maintained by a Master-sentiment. What more comprehensive sentiment can there be than the religious sentiment? What other sentiment can make it possible for us to live in our two-dimensional world? But it needs cultivation, and cannot be left to the mercy of sporadic feelings. If character depends on the organization of moral habits[1] surely our religious life will be as dependent on the organization of spiritual habits.

We have now seen that psychopathology, psychotherapy and Pastoral Psychology are closely linked together; and that all three are dependent on general psychology for their knowledge of psychological processes. Each in turn may make a contribution to general psychology. Psychopathology and psychotherapy are almost entirely concerned with mental processes which lead to personality- and character-disturbances. Pastoral Psychology, however, although it takes account of the causative factors of disturbance laid bare by psychopathology, and of methods of dealing with the mind evolved by psychotherapy, is more concerned with the mental processes of the spiritual and moral life. It alone sees man as a whole, as a soul, as a spirit whose chief end is to enjoy God. Every psychogenic disturbance it would say is to be explained ultimately in terms of a failure on the part of the individual to reach that end, that is to say, to reach a meaning to life which gives him a sense of security, takes away the feeling of aloneness, and integrates his interior life. One may put it another way and say that every neurotic trouble is due to the fact that the individual has failed to achieve a spiritual life, to be at home in the spiritual dimension of his being. The psychotherapist is not required to assign moral responsibility

1 William James, *Essay on Habit.*

to the individual for his trouble. Pastoral Psychology, on the other hand, lays great stress on the elicitation of moral responsibility and strives to deepen the sense of it. It does not deny the distinction between moral disease and sin. It would accept Dr. Hadfield's distinction[1] that moral disease is due to repressed complexes and sin to wrong sentiments ; but it would stress the fact that complexes themselves are due in many cases to a weakness of character-structure ; or, if we put it another way, to a weak self that is unwilling to integrate its impulses, ideas and desires. Character, as James Ward taught us, can only be predicated of a self, and not of that which they have in common, such as instinctive tendencies, physiological drives or sentiments. After all, as Professor Laird[2] has pointed out, instincts and sentiments can only solicit the self ; they cannot coerce it. Whereas psychotherapists speak of a re-education of disturbing mental processess Pastoral Psychology would say that unification of the mental processes can follow only after the self is master of its own house. It would deepen the consciousness of the self, its attitude to life, and to its own behaviour-tendencies. Indeed, I am not sure but that it could say with scientific accuracy that neurotic disease is due to the fact that the self, in its effort towards integration, and to preserve what integration it has achieved, refuses to integrate behaviour-tendencies which would upset its moral organization.

Not a little psychopathology could give grounds for that last sentence. There are many cases of anxiety and phobias due to the repression of behaviour-tendencies which, if expressed, would be shown to be criminal or perversions. The obsessions and compulsions have invariably repressed resentment with allied destructive tendencies. Some unadjusted lives are due to the fact that certain behaviour-tendencies

---

[1] *Psychology of Morals.*
[2] *A Study in Moral Theory,* page 138.

4

have never become mature. It is a great mistake to think that behaviour-tendencies which are repressed are different in kind from the normal impulses of which we may be conscious every day of our lives. The impulses and emotions which lie behind our normal temptations and which lead to the " seven deadly sins " of moral theology, are the same impulses lying behind a very great deal of neurosis. It is not the behaviour-tendencies which cause neurotic disease, but the repression of them, as I have emphasized. Once repression has taken place the behaviour-tendencies can ramify like a fungus, as Freud has pointed out ;[1] and they can give an illusory idea of their strength.

It might be asked here : why not eliminate the psycho-therapist ? Why not turn all these people over to the pastor ? Two things have to be noted as to why this is impossible :

First, the pastor as pastor, the Gospel as Gospel, can only deal with what is conscious, or at least not too severely repressed. The person suffering from psychological disorder differs from the person who is suffering consciously the same conflicts. The former is pre-occupied with his symptoms and almost not at all with the hidden conflict ; the latter is concerned to control the offending behaviour-tendencies. The former is afraid to be free, that is to say, to allow the offending tendencies to come into consciousness ; he dare not allow this freedom of access to the conscious mind of behaviour-tendencies because of the guilt-feelings attached to them, or because he is afraid he will not be able to control them. The mere mention of religion to some of these unfortunate victims of repression accentuates their guilt-feelings, and hence their symptoms and distress. It is this " sense of guilt ", the " conviction of sin ", as the pastor calls it, which these people fear and not the behaviour-tendencies which give rise to the sense of guilt and fear. The pastor is associated with the

[1] Sigmund Freud. *A General Selection*, page 102.

thing they fear. Hence the tendency of many to seek the psychotherapist and not the pastor. Even when they seek the pastor's help the sense of guilt which they feel is already displaced upon incidents and memories which have little or nothing to do with what is repressed, or are so trivial that one knows that the " sins " they confess could not bear the burden of anxiety and guilt-feelings experienced.

This unconscious refusal to deal with the offending impulses and ideas which they generate, is shown in another curious phenomenon. Every neurotic patient comes to analysis with two contradictory tendencies—one is to get rid of the guilt, which to them means getting better ; and the other the hope that somehow the analyst will be able to effect a lessening of the guilt or the symptoms without modifying the offending impulses lying behind the trouble. There is invariably in the neurotic this wish to indulge without the sense of guilt,[1] or anxiety or phobia symptoms. Hence it has been well said :   " The wish for recovery contains a wish for the satisfaction of the instincts as well as a wish for frustration."[2]

By way of illustration here is a case sent to me recently, one of the victims of war conditions. She is a young girl of twenty-two years of age. She complains of a pain in the breast, one in the groin, stomach upset, inflamed tongue and the inside of her cheek. She is sleepless, restless, cannot concentrate and has violent feelings. She went into the forces at eighteen. She was seduced by a married man who " packed her up " after he had given her Gonorrhoea. That had been entirely cleared up ; but she was obsessed with the idea that the poison had got into her system and was the cause of the other troubles. She was very anxious that I should recommend her going from home.

Analysis quickly showed that she had been keeping

---

[1] Stekel. *Conditions of Nervous Anxiety,* page 10.
[2] *Psycho-analysis To-day.* Edited by Sandor Lonard, page 61.

company with another married man who was separated from his wife. Seduction had again taken place, and this man was trying to persuade her to bear a child as he thought that might induce his wife to divorce him. That the girl had repressed the idea of the mess she had made of her life was obvious from various symptoms, such as the fact that she had great difficulty in swallowing. In her unconscious, she really could not swallow the life she was heading for. That, however, was perfectly unconscious. She was anxious to get rid of her symptoms and back to where this man was stationed.

Another interesting illustration is that of a man who could not go out alone, and who was pre-occupied with marriage from morning to night. Every intimation of a marriage in the newspapers of anyone he knew sent him into violent tempers. Analysis showed that he had been the victim of masturbation since his early teens. He felt ill on the emergence of guilt-feelings regarding this. Instead, however, of dealing with the habit he tried to repress it; he was unable; so his mind begins to work out how he could get the pleasure without the guilt. Married people do not have guilt about these relations. Hence there is set up in his mind a compulsive tendency to get a wife—any woman would do, he felt and indeed said. Hence the obsession in regard to marriage and his pathological envy of married people; hence, too, his fear of going out alone. His commonsense told him that not all marriages were happy; that they must be based upon something far more solid than sex relations. To save himself from an intolerable marriage he simply has to withdraw from contact.

The two illustrations show clearly the contradictory tendencies in the neurotic and why the pastor or the Gospel cannot deal with such people. To get these tendencies conscious and to help the patient to deal with them is the outcome of long analytic work. An expert knowledge of the intricacy of mental process is necessary, as well as a purely objective standpoint in regard to what the pastor would call " sin ". The pastor's exhortation to trust God when the anxiety symptoms are severe cannot operate for the simple reason that the tendencies in relation to which the anxiety or guilt-feelings are generated are hidden from consciousness.

The second reason why the pastor cannot displace the psychotherapist I have already given ; but it will not be irrelevant to give it in the words of the Rev. H. J. S. Guntripp, B.A., B.D., Lecturer in Psychology in Relation to Medicine at Leeds University School. " The whole field of psychiatry ", he says, " includes large areas that a non-medical man cannot enter in the nature of the case, such as the constitutional and organic basis of personality, technique of a physio-therapeutic kind, the psychoses of insanities, and conditions bordering on them. Medical psychology must include all that, and in my judgment the decision as to what kind of treatment any case of mental disturbance should have must rest with the psychiatrist, i.e. a doctor who is a specialist in psychological medicine. Only after that may some type of treatment, such as analysis, be carried out by the non-medical psychologist, if such treatment is appropriate."[1]

Mr. Guntripp is far from belittling the capacity of Pastoral Psychology to co-operate with medicine ; he urges it for a wide field. He recognizes " that much vague and specific ill-health is traceable to unhappiness, emotional stress, to social maladjustment and to unfortunate character-formations. The problems of neurosis ", he concludes, " are often exaggerations of the problems common to us all."

The last sentence really gives the field of Pastoral Psychology—" the problems common to us all ". Neuroses, apart from the constitutional and organic, arise in the manner

[1] Carr's Lane Congregational Church Magazine, March, 1944.

we meet the common problems of life, the crises through which we all pass. Our reaction to these crises, our manner of dealing with them lay down a pre-disposition which issues in a character-formation or trend. Many of the situations to which we respond in the wrong way should never arise and are due to environmental pressures. Nevertheless, there is no psychological situation until there is a response, and it is the response which is vital. Other situations arise with the development of personality itself. Again these problems are common to us all. Thus we can make the generalization that character-disturbance, whether it issues in the neuroses or not, is determined by the manner in which the individual reacts to his problems.

To understand more deeply the reactions of the individual to the problems common to us all, we must now study the mental processes involved. The terms " repression " and the " unconscious ", as well as numerous other processes, must be accurately elucidated. Once we understand these processes we can conclude with a study of the nature and origin of conflicts and their resolution.

MENTAL MECHANISMS

It is almost impossible to over-estimate the tremendous advance in our knowledge of behaviour-tendencies that came with the concepts of the "unconscious" and "repression". Without an understanding of these concepts it is not possible to be otherwise than bewildered at the vagaries and irrationality of human beings, whether neurotic or not. When you listen to an apparently religious person telling you that he has an almost irresistible desire to swear at God, or to a young girl who wants to say her prayers to the devil, or to a clever, intelligent business man that he cannot go to bed if there is a poker in the room, or to a woman who loves her child that she has a compulsion to throw the child out of the window, or to another who said that when she was out walking in the streets she had the feeling that she was not walking on the pavement but on a level with the house-tops, you begin to think that you have entered a more unexpected world than that of "Alice in Wonderland".

These are simple examples compared with the distressing symptoms of neurotic disease, or with irrational character-disturbances. It was on all these irrationalities that Freud threw light by his concepts of the "unconscious" and "repression". These are not easy concepts to understand ; unless, as Dr. Wm. Brown has said, one has undergone some kind of analysis or attempted to analyse someone else.

It is true that the concept of the unconscious was discussed long before Freud. Leibnitz and Hartmann both made use of the idea of the unconscious. Leibnitz maintained that the facts of mental life are unintelligible unless we assume that in the mental sphere tendencies are present and active

45

whose degree of consciousness is " infinitesimal ".   Hartmann thought that all impressions which disappear from the conscious, leave traces or dispositions which are essentially physical and not mental at all.   Professor William James thought he had found in the concept of the unconscious an explanation of our inactive memories, our obscurely motived passions, our likes and dislikes, our prejudices and preferences. He thought also that it was the source of our dreams.

Whatever contribution we may think any of these made to our understanding of mental process and the continuity of interest as well as the unity of the mind, it must be to Freud that we turn if we desire to understand the relation of the unconscious to behaviour, especially of an abnormal kind. It is to him, in the first place, that we owe the concept of repression, the process by which what we are experiencing remains or is made unconscious.

The meaning of both these concepts still remains confused even in writers whose lucidity on other questions no one could deny.[1]   As I have already remarked, unless one does some analysis on one's self and in a sense catches the process in the act the actual knowledge of the unconscious and repression eludes us.

We shall first consider repression, for this is the process by which the unconscious becomes unconscious.   It may be defined as that process whereby we are prevented from perceiving some activity of the mind, such as a character-trait, or a motive, or the meaning of a behaviour-tendency.   Through repression the normal process of perception of external objects may become disturbed and distorted.   I had a young man whose complaint was that his nose had a habit of swelling and becoming very red.   Recently I had a woman who was in a state of agitated anxiety, and the reason she gave was that

---

[1] Cf. McKenzie. *Psychology, Psycho-therapy and Evangelicalism,* pages 88ff.

her face had become ugly by the presence of growing hairs. The young man had just an ordinary nose on the snubby side ; while the woman was fair and not a dark hair was to be seen on her face.

Many people confuse " repression " with " suppression ". Dr. Rivers did not use the term " repress ", but spoke of " witting " and " unwitting " suppression. His " unwitting suppression " is equivalent to the meaning of " repression ". When we speak of a child being repressed we really mean that it is suppressed by its parents or teachers ; its initiative and individuality are in danger, and the child has found it easier to become submissive. This leads to repression on the part of the child. Repression in an inward or, if I may use the jargon, " endo-psychic " process. No one can " repress " us ; but we can be " suppressed ". Probably Rivers thought that " repressed " behaviour-tendencies or emotions were conscious at one time and then wittingly repressed, until the process became automatic and unconscious.

Repression must be clearly differentiated from suppression. Repression is a refusal to perceive something active in the mind. It is, as Dr. David Yellowlees has put it, " a refusal to see ",[1] not a refusal to do. It is unconscious. Suppression is a perfectly conscious process ; it is a refusal to put some idea into action ; it is a conscious restraint of impulse or emotion. Repression is the unconscious process whereby we prevent some tendency active in the mind from becoming conscious ; suppression is the conscious prevention of a tendency from expressing itself after it has entered consciousness.

Suppose someone calls when we are in the midst of a meal, or on the point of running to an appointment. Naturally we feel annoyed. Convention, our professional conscience, or some other motive, may require us to hide our feelings of annoyance, even to look pleased. In temptation

[1] Cf. Stekel. *Conditions of Anxiety,* page 6.

we are perfectly conscious of some tendency soliciting our attention and urging us to some act ; consciously we suppress the tendency. In repression we are not aware of the tendency, motive or emotion excluded from consciousness.

The suppressed or repressed tendency, however, reaches consciousness in one form or another. Our annoyance at the inconvenient visit may show itself in little restless movements, in the tone of our voice, or we may find ourselves being over-polite. If the behaviour-tendency is unacceptable to our self-respect and we repress it, it will manifest itself in some kind of a neurotic symptom such as a phobia, an anxiety-state, guilt-feelings or depression, or it may be in some kind of irrational behaviour, or a physical symptom.

Illustration is better than abstract definitions. Here is a man who all his life has thought himself to be religious in a quiet deep way. Suddenly he finds himself with a tendency to utter blasphemous words regarding God. He tends also to be pre-occupied with little bodily symptoms. The resentment first showed itself when he was recovering from influenza. He was lying in the garden on a couch and his wife came and was arranging the rugs when the words compulsively entered his mind. Analysis showed a compulsive tendency to restrict his desires within narrow limits. Apparently he had submitted to his religious ideals but had never assimilated them. In his unconscious he resented the restrictions, and the repressed resentment comes up in the compulsive swear words against God.

Thus, when we repress anything active in the mind we do not destroy it, nor modify it ; it remains dynamic and is continually striving for an entrance to consciousness.

This will be better understood through a grasp of the concept of the " unconscious ".

The difficulty regarding the acceptance of this concept is only possible to those who equate consciousness with mind, or conscious with " mental ". The latter term is much wider than consciousness or conscious. There can be no question of the fact that there are mental processes which must be active before we are aware of them. Impressions upon our sense organs do not always become conscious although if we were to attend to them undoubtedly we should be conscious of them. If I draw my hand over the hairs of my other hand I shall be conscious of the sensation arising from their movement ; but normally I do not notice these. The threshold of consciousness or awareness is the term used to denote the degree of impression upon a sense organ before we become aware of the sensation. But the threshold is dependent on other things than the impression. Custom can heighten the threshold, as, for example, in those living near a railway line ; they will scarcely notice the noise of a passing train. The mind tends to keep from awareness habitual impressions which would distract it. The impression, however, must reach the brain although the mind ignores it.

A deeper degree of unconscious mental process is seen in the Laws of Association. The similarity of one person to another is not made by deliberate comparison in consciousness ; the conscious mind simply becomes aware of an association already made. In other words, the Laws of Association bring together ideas and emotions in a region beyond consciousness ; we become aware of the connection after it is already made in the subconscious region. We become aware of ideas ; we do not think them. They are instruments we use to think by. We can compare ideas ; we can reflect upon them ; we can draw conclusions from them ; but we do not think them.

We get deeper still when we speak of an " unconscious wish ". We must not confuse " wish " with " desire ". A desire, as Hobhouse writes, is " the idea of an anticipated end ". It is perfectly conscious. The " wish " in the sense of an unconscious wish has no conscious anticipation of its

49

end. The "wish" is simply a mental process pushing towards consciousness where it would appear with a certain amount of attractiveness in the same way as our temptations appear to us. In temptation we "wish" what we do not desire. The "wish" has a certain amount of compulsiveness which a normal desire has not, as, for example, the swear words of the patient already mentioned, which appear as an urge to utter them. Sometimes "unconscious wish" is used as synonymous with "unconscious motive".

The question has been raised and has given a great deal of difficulty to some writers, as to whether the "unconscious wish" has any unconscious ideational content. Is the idea of the end-action part of the unconscious process? Mr. Mellone is representative of many who contend that unconscious ideational content is "nonsense". He writes, "We must beware of speaking of 'an unconscious idea' or an 'unconscious wish' and the like. Strictly speaking, any such expression is nonsense. It is like speaking of 'an unconscious conscious process'. It is admissable only if understood as 'verbal shorthand'. An 'unconscious idea' or 'wish' is a mental process which manifests itself in consciousness or if it could manifest itself in consciousness, would produce some idea, desire or emotion as the case may be. Such a process is conveniently termed a 'psychological disposition'." He comes hard up against the late Professor William James for speaking of a " set of memories, thoughts and feelings which are outside the primary consciousness, but yet must be classed as conscious facts of some sort, able to reveal their presence by unmistakable signs ". " James ", he says, " was fond of 'slapdash' expressions and the description of these processes as conscious is an example. He should, of course, have said, 'mental facts'." James is asserting ideational content to these facts; and Mr. Mellone is failing to take account of facts which James must have considered.

When we are asleep we are unconscious or we seem to be. Nevertheless when a person talks in his sleep he is expressing ideas, and fulfilling "unconscious wishes". In sleep we are in touch with nothing but mental processes. A sleep-walker acts as if his actions were guided by the idea of an end. Moreover, the mind must somehow be conscious of the end-action towards which an unconscious wish moves, else how can we explain the anxiety and the fact that we repress the "wish". The anxiety in consciousness is not referred to this end-action, and indeed may be displaced on to something that should cause no anxiety at all. The process has meaning to the mind before we become conscious of the process at all. Ideas, as we have seen, are not conscious productions; we become aware of them already in our minds.

No one more than the psychotherapist is aware of the difficulties of the problem of the ideational content of the unconscious wish or motive. One psychotherapist has suggested that the "unconscious wish" or idea works more like a "conditioned reflex" than a deliberate judgment. We do know that the unconscious seems to be unoriented in regard to time and place as well as reality.

Take an illustration. I had a woman sent to me by her doctor who was full of apprehensiveness and anxiety. She had not long been out of the hospital where she had an operation on the fallopian tubes so as to prevent conception. She had one child, and the birth was so difficult that she was warned to have no more children. After a lapse of eleven years she became pregnant; as soon as she knew she became very distressed. The pregnancy was terminated, and the operation performed successfully, and during her stay in the hospital she was perfectly free from anxiety. Immediately she met her husband on the doorstep of her home the anxiety began again and became intense. The unconscious fear of pregnancy was as active as if she had not undergone an operation at all. Such a situation-neurosis is comparatively easy to clear up ; but it is difficult not to believe that the idea of pregnancy was in her mind ; because one can only have fear if the situation has some meaning for one. The idea of danger must somewhere be present else there is no fear.

Actually there is no mental process which does not involve cognition, conation and emotion. One or other of these moments of the process may be more prominent than the others ; but the whole three are involved. My position is that the " unconscious wish " or " motive " is exactly what a conscious wish or motive is except that it lacks awareness. Mind is a far wider term than consciousness. That does not mean to say that awareness or consciousness is not exceedingly important for personal life. On the contrary, it is of the utmost importance. Only as mental process becomes conscious are we able to modify it, and to direct it towards ends consistent with the ends of personality itself. The unconscious seems to have little power of discrimination. Neurotic affection, e.g. or a neurotic tendency to restrict one's desires and wishes, can always be differentiated from the normal tendency to affection or to self-control of our desires by the fact that the former is always indiscriminate. The individual with a neurotic need for approval compulsively seeks the approval of people whose opinions do not matter a scrap. A man with neurotic hostility is perfectly unreasonable in regard to what he gets into a violent temper for. Consciousness or awareness is vitally important. Someone has said that anyone who has increased our consciousness of self has made a contribution to progress. That I think is true in the sense that to the degree we have the capacity to perceive the processes motivating our behaviour to that degree we are able to unify the self.

Probably we should not draw a hard and fast line between conscious and unconscious. It is possible to state the problem in terms of degrees of consciousness or awareness of mental processes. Some motives of behaviour we seem able to perceive without let or hindrance. There are others, however, whose meaning we resist although they are obvious enough to outsiders. An individual will go on dodging every difficult situation; he can always provide "good" reasons for his avoidance of what he ought to have seen. Once, however, he has become aware of his tendency to dodge or shirk responsibility, he can look back and *know* that he has always been a shirker. Resistance is set up in the mind against unwelcome truth. That repression is the outcome of resistance to insight we know from the fact that immediately we try to make the individual aware of his motives or the meaning of his actions we are met with strong opposition. Every patient or individual difficult to get on with suffers because he resists the meanings of his own behaviour which are often as plain as a pike-staff to others who have no special knowledge of psychology. It is not the lack of intelligence, nor the capacity for insight that neurotics lack. More often than not they are above the average. They refuse to become aware, they refuse to perceive their own mental processes.

We begin to see an answer to the question of Professor Holt: "Why is the Unconscious Unconscious?" In the more distressing cases with which the psychotherapist or psychiatrist deals we can say that the unconscious contains some threat to their moral integrity, or to the conception they have of themselves. We all have a mask with which we present ourselves to the outside world and even to ourselves. We have a tendency to believe that the masks we wear are really indicative of what we are in reality, and we tend to inhibit everything that would contradict our belief. It is not easy for one to acknowledge to himself that he is envious, or proud, or lustful, or hostile. Some have tendencies which, if they were allowed to enter consciousness, would create an almost unbearable sense of insecurity ; others have tendencies which, if they become conscious, would at once disturb their personal relationships. We have a wonderful capacity for thinking that we are cleverer and better than we are ; and probably without this capacity we should be unable to face life at all. I cannot agree with Jung's statement that the unconscious is always the antithesis of the conscious ; the generalization is too wide. There can be no question, however, that it applies to all the severe cases of neuroticism. We are, as a matter of fact, often better than we think we are. Many people who have no connection with the Church, and indeed would repudiate a religious motive, are sustained in their moral lives and in their good works by a religious sentiment which for one reason or another is not allowed to function in consciousness. That sentiment motivates them more than they realize or would acknowledge.

It is not always the unconscious pretence that we are better than we are that causes us to repress or to keep from awareness tendencies which are active in our mind and behaviour. There is no feeling so unbearable, either in a child or an adult, than the feeling of insecurity. The Behaviourists contend that one of the innate fears in the infant is roused by a sense of insecurity. Hold an infant in such a way that it feels physically insecure and at once the child will show all the signs of fear. A sudden loud noise is the other stimulus to innate fear according to the same school of thought.

A sense of psychological insecurity in the child creates not fear but anxiety. As the child grows older the anxiety can stimulate the imagination and the imagination can conjure up all sorts of fearsome objects as the cause of the anxiety. A child needs affection and anything that causes the child to feel insecure regarding the affection of the parents is not seldom the beginning of neuroticism, or of character-trends which may play a vital part in the child's reactions to life in general. A home where the parents show to each other violent tempers and in their quarrels speak in a loud voice leaves inevitably a sense of insecurity in most children. The threatening father or mother whose crossness gives the child a feeling that the parent's love may be withdrawn at any moment compels the child to react in some way by which it will regain its sense of security, and stave off the hostile feelings of the parent. The child tends to repress the sense of insecurity and anxiety. Because it cannot bear not to be loved, because it is afraid of hostile feelings on the part of others, the child resorts to repression and the conscious is made unconscious. Whatever hostile feelings the behaviour of the parents arouse in the child may be feebly expressed by the child at first, but the fear of the parents' reaction to its hostility soon makes the child repress the hostile feelings felt within itself. It may then develop a tendency to be submissive with the hostility repressed.

The sense of insecurity, however, may not be in relation to the parents or the outside world; the child may feel threatened from within its own mind. At the beginning of his volume on the *Two Sources of Morality and Religion* Bergson speaks of that period of life when the child is untrammelled by any moral inhibitions. Then comes the day when the child's moral life opens with a prohibition from within. What happens is that the prohibitions of the parents or teachers are introjected by the child. The moral control, once exerted externally by parents and teachers, now works from within the child's own mind. In the child the conscience is for the most part prohibitive and compulsive. It exercises itself as a " must " or " must not ". If the child has not done something it feels it ought to have done, or done something which it knows the parents would disapprove or what at some time has been prohibited, guilt-feelings arise,

55

5A

and may become very strong. Guilt-feelings always contain a threat, and the threat may be projected by the child upon something external. Hence the irrational fears of the dark. The fear of these guilt-feelings will make the child cling more closely to the parent. If the guilt-feelings are associated with behaviour-tendencies of the child it may repress the behaviour-tendencies, and then it gets a feeling of insecurity from two sides: on the one hand, from the guilt-feelings, and on the other, from the behaviour-tendencies.

This negative conscience[1] is what in psycho-analytic theory is called the " super-ego "; what I have myself called the "infantile conscience". It is always either prohibitive or compulsive. In psycho-analytic theory the term is designed to convey the idea that superimposed upon the child's ego are the teachings of parents and teachers. Their teachings and what the child senses from the moral atmosphere becomes the "ego-ideal". The child is compelled to live up to this ego-ideal, by inward compulsion. The super-ego is thus the guardian of this ego-ideal; it restrains the child from doing anything contrary to its imperatives.

It is not, in my opinion, equivalent to conscience. The developed conscience is always positive. The conscience is that principle which co-ordinates and regulates our behaviour-tendencies according to the ideals we have consciously or unconsciously accepted. Its content has been assimilated, not merely introjected. To that content the mature mind has a spontaneous relation. It becomes the guide to action, and contains the standard of moral judgment by which the mind judges spontaneously as to what is right and wrong, good or bad, just or unjust. The negative or infantile conscience is entirely prohibitive and compulsive. The positive conscience is integrated with the rest of the personality; the

[1] Cf. *Psychology, Psycho-therapy and Evangelicalism.* Chapter on " Prolegomena to Religious Experience ".

prohibitive conscience lies over against the behaviour-tendencies as though it were external to the child. When the prohibitive conscience is disobeyed guilt-feelings arise ; when we have come below our positive ideals we experience shame.

Our moral education, thus, begins with prohibitions and I doubt if it could begin in any other way. The child is not of an age when it can perceive the reasons for right or wrong, good or bad. It has to be restrained from many actions not because they are wrong but because they might lead to danger of either a physical or moral kind. There are " musts " and " must nots " in the training of a child in cleanliness, moral habits and manners. Every prohibition carries an implicit threat of some evil consequence if the direction is disobeyed. Some activities of the child may lead to moral habits difficult to break ; its impulses, especially its sex impulses, may get an outlet in a wrong direction. Parents and teachers react very differently to a child who has been caught slapping another child, or who has taken another child's toy, and to the same child if caught in any form of sexual play or indulging in some form of bodily pleasure. They convey to the child a sense of guilt towards anything sexual which makes a strong impression on the child's mind. If the guilt is associated with punishments of God the child may grow up with a distorted conception of God, one in which God becomes an outsize of the threatening parent. That means almost irreparable damage ; and the prohibitive conscience is likely to remain. The child grows up fearing evil rather than loving good ; afraid of vice rather than in love with virtue. To the degree the parents elicit guilt-feelings to that degree the child grows up with a feeling of insecurity : it feels insecure in the presence of the guilt-feelings ; and insecure in regard to the behaviour-tendencies whose activity tends to arouse the guilt-feelings. To propitiate its own infantile conscience the child may resort to self-punishment ; to avoid the temptation of the behaviour-tendencies, the child may repress them.

Naturally the psycho-analyst has paid more attention to the super-ego than the positive conscience. He is concerned with the guilt-feelings with which his patients are so burdened. To have drawn the attention to these guilt-feelings as moments in the downward thrust of repression is to have drawn attention to what is unhealthy, and is a real contribution to the problem as to why the unconscious is unconscious.

The repression of behaviour-tendencies is the unconscious attempt to avoid the sense of insecurity coming from these tendencies and also the attempt to avoid the guilt-feelings. Alas ; the guilt-feelings are seldom repressed ; as a rule they are displaced. But the presence of guilt-feelings is invariably a sign that the offending behaviour-tendencies are active in the unconscious.

For Pastoral Psychology the light thrown upon this infantile conscience is exceedingly important. Guilt-feelings are always morbid ; the healthy reaction to wrong-doing is repentance, which includes both sorrow for our wrong-doing and the modifying of the offending tendencies. The pastor should not attempt to arouse guilt-feelings ; his work is to stimulate the positive conscience. Guilt-feelings inevitably alienate the soul from God ; and they often generate violent feelings of defiance against God or religion in general. A healthy sense of shame and humility at our weaknesses just as inevitably deepens and strengthens our relationship to God.

A word on moral education is not irrelevant here. Unfortunately our education in morality is apt to emphasize these prohibitions ; and sometimes the child's moral education is nothing but prohibitions. Many wise parents and teachers, however, are more concerned that the child should love the good rather than hate evil, that he should cultivate virtue rather than avoid vice, and great care is taken to associate the child's behaviour-tendencies with what brings approval. As the child's capacity for moral insight develops he begins to see one activity as better than another. The result is that the morally well-educated child tends to leave the prohibitions behind, and his behaviour-tendencies instead of being restrained by threats of disapproval from without or within are guided spontaneously by the child's growing sense of rightness and wrongness. These are the children who grow up to be what Professor William James called "the once born". They have no threatening conscience; no sense of alienation from God, parents or teachers. The conscience grows more and more informed, and instead of being like the super-ego or prohibitive conscience, an internalized policeman, it becomes a spontaneous guide and inspiration to the growing personality.

Nevertheless, the prohibitive conscience never disappears. It has an adult function. In the adult it exercises restraint; not the restraint that is re-enforced by fear, but a restraint that induces reflection on any contemplated activity. It still condemns wrong-doing, but not through the repressing factors of fear and guilt, but through a healthy shame and humility which leads to a spontaneous correction of the faults. Theology would do well to take account of this fact in its theories of the Atonement. Many of these theories embody the threats and penalties of the prohibitive conscience; and these get projected upon God.

The development of the Christian adult conscience would take a series of lectures in itself. Here we are only concerned with the perversion of conscience. It is to this perversion of conscience or to the confusion of the prohibitive conscience with the adult conscience that we must look for the roots of rigoristic ethics, the doctrine of eternal punishment, religious scrupulosity and the penal theories of the Atonement. The prohibitive conscience keeps the religious soul under Law, as

St. Paul found, instead of under grace ; it makes duty a burden to carry instead of the dynamic direction of behaviour-tendencies. The perfect contrast between the life ruled by the prohibitive conscience and that ruled by the positive conscience is implicit in St. Paul's chapter on Love. Most of the types of conversion familiar to us from Professor William James and other books are conversions from a prohibitive conscience to a positive Christian one.

It must be noted that the prohibitive conscience can be repressed instead of left behind, and always with baneful results. If it is perfectly repressed we get the rather truculent individual who can say : " Evil be thou my good " without turning a hair, or without sign of a nervous symptom. If the repression is not too successful we get certain types of neurotic trouble such as anxiety-states, melancholia, or paranoiac symptoms. Whether it is consciously active or repressed the prohibitive conscience, in my opinion, is the greatest disturber of the mental, moral and spiritual life.

A good deal of the answer to the question as to why the unconscious is unconscious will be found in the concept of the prohibitive conscience or super-ego. The ego becomes afraid of the guilt-feelings ; it is continually bombarded by threats, by anxiety, fear ; and the function of these threats, etc., is to dare the ego to indulge in the prohibited tendencies, or even to allow them into consciousness. It is not the whole answer to the question, however, as we have seen.

There is a law of attention which might be formulated thus : Any tendency active in the mind tends to inhibit anything that would distract the attention from it ; and to bring into consciousness everything that would keep the attention focused upon it. When we are repressing anything the subconscious mind is pre-occupied in keeping that some-thing out of consciousness, and brings into consciousness what is likely to keep the attention away from the repressed elements. Hence a pre-occupation with guilt-feelings will tend to keep out of the mind behaviour-tendencies to which the guilt-feelings are attached ; a subconscious pre-occupation with the sense of insecurity will bring into consciousness anything that will give us a sense of security.

Although I have spoken of repression as though it were an impersonal process we must not be misled by the necessities of formulation. The process is an activity of the self ; it is the self acting, as it were, in self-defence. The self is guarding its own integrity ; it is attempting to control its own behaviour-tendencies ; or to avoid insights which would cause painful emotions. The self turns away from its own content.

All this leads to a further question : How does the self manage to keep from consciousness what is unacceptable ? How does it keep its own tendencies from reaching consciousness ? How can I manage to deny the pride in me which others see so plainly ? Or the envy that makes me jealous and which manifests itself so obviously to other people ? How can I fail to see that my " love " is ego-centric, childish, selfish and nothing more than a means to ulterior ends ; and how do I manage to deny it to myself when others tell me that it is so ?

It seems a wild hypothesis to premise that the ego can hide from itself its motives, the meaning of its acts, its lusts and hates. Yet it is so. Actions whose meaning is perfectly clear to everyone else we account for in such a way as to justify them to our own minds at least, or to deny to ourselves their motives. We unconsciously resist the meaning to our own acts which we unhesitatingly would give to the same acts if we saw them in someone else. The inner perceptive process is distorted, or refused entrance to consciousness by an elaborate system of defence mechanisms. These defence mechanisms are designed not only to deceive others but ourselves.

The most familiar of these mechanisms is known as *Rationalization*. *It may be defined as the giving to ourselves " good" reasons, not the " real" reasons, for what we think, feel or do.* Our intellectual processes are perverted in the interests of the hidden motives. A man will give elaborate reasons as to why he should not obey the conventions, or the rules of a society or club ; he will overlook the fact that no society can be run without conventions of some sort, or a club without rules any more than the traffic could run smoothly in our streets without a law of the road. Underneath he is a rebel to all rules and authority ; and that fact he represses.

Rationalizations may be used in the interests of some gratification which the individual refuses to acknowledge he desires or wishes. The thing to note here is that rationalization is not making an excuse, is not telling a deliberate lie, no more than psychological illness is malingering. The rationalization is made with conviction, a conviction not very easy to undermine.

A woman came to me some time ago telling me that she had an almost irresistible desire to join the Roman Catholic Church. She gave a dozen arguments for doing so. When we got down to the real reasons I found that she had become infatuated with another woman who was her superior in business ; and the neurotic need for approval and to be liked, had forced her to "believe" that she desired earnestly to change her religious convictions. The woman whose "love" she wanted was a Roman Catholic and a strong proselytizer. The patient had been sufficiently analysed before to recognize the possibility of the unconscious motive. A little later, when the proselytizer saw that she was not gong to make a proselyte, she turned against the patient ; and instead of the infatuation and the neurotic compulsion to get this woman's love at any price, there took its place unreasonable hate.

Such a process can be seen at its best in those with a neurotic tendency to evade responsibilities. The dodger can give a dozen reasons for evading what anyone could see was his duty. Neurotic anxiety can be made to look like a very honest and straightforward fear by rationalization. Karen Horney instances the over-solicitous mother who suffers from a neurotic need for affection. Such a mother will go to any lengths of sacrifice and care to protect her child from this disease or that. If she is told that she is really rationalizing she will energetically " prove " the possibility of this disease or that, this accident or that.

The hypochondriac can produce rationalizations for his imagined illnesses quicker than the psychotherapist can refute them. The paranoiac can give an elaborate argument for his delusions. One of the best examples is given by Bernhard Hart in his small but excellent volume on *Psychology of Insanity*. Here was a lad who could debate with keen skill and marshalled arguments against orthodox Christianity. The real reason for his doubts, and the motive behind the amount of energy and thought he had put into his reading was the fact that a fellow Sunday School teacher had run off with his girl. His resentment was repressed ; he apparently did not care. The resentment was hidden by being turned against their religion.

Anyone, however, with a little capacity to be honest with himself will find a multitude of examples in himself probably on any day of the week. It is a process which we all use when our motives are shady, or not altogether above board. Let a man forget his wife's birthday, or their marriage day, and when challenged he is likely to make a good rationalization ; he is not very willing to admit that we only forget what we don't want to remember.

Projection is the method of defence reaction by which we hide from ourselves our unconscious tendencies. *We may*

63

define it as the process whereby the individual who is unable to repress the ideas or tendencies within himself thrusts them into the minds of others. The person unable to approve of himself consciously will project upon another what really is self-criticism. In this way he is able to abuse his own faults without having to reproach himself. The husband or wife who feels insecure in loyalty to his or her partner will often accuse the other of adultery. I have seen many cases of this type and only in one of them did I find the accusations true. Here it was not so much an accusation as a fear that the partner might do it again. In all the others I found that the promiscuous tendencies were in the accuser ; one had been keeping a mistress for five years ! The shirker has a wonderful capacity to see his colleagues dodging their responsibilities ; the lazy individual can orate against laziness much better than the diligent, busy bee. I have seen those who have lost the capacity for self-control of their impulses and emotions project their lack of discipline upon the children they were teaching in school.

Unfortunately, projection does not lessen our anxiety ; on the contrary, it tends to increase it. When we refuse to face self-criticism we may tend to project in such a way that we act in other people's company as though they knew what we think or feel in our unconscious.

The purpose of projection is to defend us against the pain of admitting to ourselves tendencies which we would be compelled to condemn in others. Let us tend to get angry in a discussion and before we know what we are doing we are accusing our opponent of heat and partiality. We frequently project in dreams. The girl who wants men to run after her almost invariably has dreams of being chased. Hostility is another tendency which is often projected. The boy with a rebel tendency is very apt to project his own hostility into his father's mind. I have seldom found fathers so harsh as children have tried to make them out to be. Actually these patients fear the hostile feelings within themselves, for as a rule they are projected upon the father against whom they are directed, and against whom hostility would be futile.

Karen Horney has drawn attention to the fact that a tendency to retaliation may get hold of the repressed hostile impulses and thus re-enforce them. The result is that " a person who wants to injure, cheat, deceive others has also a fear that they will do the same to him. How far the retaliation fear is ingrained in human nature, how far it arises from primitive experience of sin and punishment, how far it presupposes a drive for personal revenge, I leave an open question. Beyond doubt it plays a great role in the minds of neurotic persons."[1]

Displacement is another mechanism by which we can defend ourselves from the unconscious. It plays a prominent part in the minds of those who have no desire to relinquish tendencies which their own conscience would condemn. Instead of feeling guilt about something we ought to feel guilty about, we displace the guilt-feelings on to something, as a rule, less culpable than the condemned tendency. The man half afraid of his wife will displace his resentment at something she has done on his workmates or, if he happens to be an employer or foreman, on those under him. I saw a woman who nearly sent back to the university her degree because she thought she had cribbed or not played fair. As a matter of fact she was displacing guilt from something about which she ought to have felt shame upon any little thing of which there was the slightest possibility of laxity or dishonesty.

Over-compensation is another defence mechanism which can be seen in some people. We can hide our own unconscious tendencies by an over-emphasis upon their opposite. The prude is invariably troubled in her unconscious with

[1] *The Neurotic Personality of Our Time*, page 71.

uncontrolled sex tendencies. I have had the unenviable privilege of looking into the minds of some rather belligerent conscientious objectors. In every one of them I found very strong rebel tendencies with strong hostile feelings these latter were repressed. Others I have seen who were really afraid of anything to do with war, acknowledged their fear and dread of entering the forces. In these individuals over-compensation or rationalization had not taken place ; but in the unconscious the hostile feelings were very strong, and it was of these they were afraid. It does not follow, of course, that logical and good grounds cannot be given for pacifism ; but there can be no doubt that in many it is an over-compensation for repressed hostile feelings of which they are afraid. The fear of not making a good impression will often make an individual over-polite or over-fussy.

A more subtle way of defending oneself against the unconscious becoming conscious is to deny the feeling of insecurity and the anxiety which it generates. This is the mechanism behind what is known as " Conversion hysteria." The anxiety and insecurity are expressed through physical symptoms. The milder symptoms such as diarrhœa or a tendency to urinate frequently, constipation, or the tendency to palpitation, may hide from consciousness that certain impulses are active in our minds. The more distressing symptoms such as functional paralysis, migraine, difficulty in walking, etc., keep entirely from consciousness the unconscious elements which cause anxiety.

In our next lecture we shall see all these tendencies fulfilling their function of keeping us unaware of character-trends of which we are unconscious.

It is these concepts and defence mechanisms which have thrown light upon all the abnormalities of behaviour of which we spoke in the opening paragraph of this lecture. Through a knowledge of these mechanisms we are able to see that the work of analysis or spiritual direction is to help people to perceive what is active in their minds, and to act according to the reality of the situation. As one has well said : " The task of therapy, generally speaking, is to mobilize the energies of the id, to make the super-ego more tolerant, and to help the ego to regain its synthetic and sublimating faculties as well as its own function of undisturbed perception and purposeful action."[1] Repression demobilizes the energy of our unconscious structure, so that it cannot be used by the conscious mind to fulfil its desires ; it also prevents the ego from synthesizing our impulses or integrating them with the rest of our personality through which their energy goes out not in crude ways but in re-enforcing our normal and legitimate interests. The unconscious has to be made conscious ; the perceptive processes must fulfil their natural function of allowing the conscious mind to become aware of what is active within the mind. As this task is fulfilled the individual loses his sense of insecurity whether that insecurity is felt in regard to the world as a whole or to the inner demands of our human nature. Until that is achieved conflict reigns within the mind ; incompatible tendencies are striving for contradictory goals. To those conflicts we must now turn our attention.

[1] *Psycho-Analysis To-day*, page 57.

THE NATURE, ORIGIN AND RESOLUTION OF CONFLICTS

WE have heard a good deal about personality-disorders, maladaptations, symptoms, and character-formations ; now we must turn and learn something about the nature and origin of the conflicts which manifest themselves in these aberrations. Every failure to reach a mature and stable personality begins in some kind of conflict.

We may define psychological conflict as *the presence in the mind of two or more dynamic tendencies striving simultaneously for incompatible goals.* We may have a strong tendency to submit to authority, and at the same time just as strong a tendency to hate and rebel against the same authority. We may have a strong tendency to keep the respect of our fellows and at the same time have a tendency to indulge in behaviour which is anti-social. If we have a hard rigorous moral ideal and at the same time strong impulses which have never been integrated with the rest of the personality, we shall experience conflict. If our sex impulses have never been integrated with a love-sentiment, and yet loyalty to marriage ideals is demanded by our conscience, the promiscuous impulses must be repressed or so rationalized as to be disguised ; in either case there will be conflict and a sense of insecurity ; probably guilt-feelings.

What we have to note is that psychological conflict is always interior ; that is, it is a conflict within the mind. The tendencies in conflict have always incompatible goals. The reaction to this conflict produces the personality-disorders ; if there is any attempt to repress the conflicting tendencies, neurotic symptoms appear and the trouble begins. It should

consciousness with the regressed energy the individual would have the feeling that he wanted to do what he did as a child.

Real conflicts, the conflicts which give the bias to character-formation begin with self-consciousness. It is then that the child becomes conscious of forbidden fruit, of prohibitions which arise from within. It is then that the child begins to react consciously to the feeling of insecurity ; for it is not till then that ·the child can experience what Eric Fromm calls " aloneness ". The child before self-consciousness may be conscious of comfortable feelings when someone is with it, or of uncomfortable feelings if alone ; but that is a different experience from " aloneness ".

It is at the dawn of self-consciousness that the child may react to the sense of insecurity by a greater leaning on the parents, or seek the shelter of friendly people. It is then also that the child may react to authority by submission rather than incur the anger of parents or teachers. It is then also that the child's curiosity can really be aroused and the child seek to formulate questions and seek information. Nor is it till then that the child experiences real guilt-feelings in the sense that it has done something reproachable. It is at this period, as far as I have gathered from my observation, that the child internalizes the prohibitions which so often pre-determine the child's moral attitudes. With these prohibitions internalized the stage is set for the interior conflicts whose repression results in neuroticism or difficulty in moral growth. Before this period the child's conflicts were with external objects, such as the parents, other children, or with materials of its play. Now the conflicts are within the child's own mind, between tendencies within itself. How the child then reacts to its problems, its attitude to them, has a strong deter-mining influence on the child's future modes of reacting to life itself and other people.

Nevertheless, it does not follow that we need to dig into the man's past until we come on these early problems before it is possible to understand and help the individual, or to show him his character-traits or his false attitudes. Patients as a rule become interested in the origin of an attitude once it is conscious, but they can become conscious of attitudes and character-traits long before they can trace their origin. The genetic approach to character-disorders is not the best approach. To help anyone we must understand what they are now, what attitudes they are exhibiting to life now when faced with definite situations. Although the origin of the attitudes lies in the first reactions to life, we can be sure that the attitude has been modified to some extent by later experience. Certainly to understand any character-formation thoroughly we must go back and study its origin or beginnings, what it was a reaction to, why the child took this particular reaction, and that will help us to understand why he is taking that attitude now in adulthood. The pre-occupation with origins, however, may make us undervalue later experiences, and keep us from assessing these early reactions at their true value. It does not correct a man's obstinacy to be told that as a child he was resentful when compelled to perform his ablutions. He can quite believe it although he can never get any knowledge of it. What he wants to know is how he can modify his compulsive obstinacy now. Most people when a character-structure has been made conscious to them recognize that they have always been so ; there is, as a rule, continuity of the tendency from self-consciousness ; but that does not help them to get rid of it now. However early the conflict arose the vital matter is that we are dealing with conflicts experienced now.

We have seen that Freud's theory of the origin of conflicts is that they are the outcome of frustrations. It is not, however, the frustration which is the causative factor. The frustration gives the child or the man the opportunity to react. The vital matter is the reaction.

We may illustrate theories about origin by examining the theory of Dr. Ian Suttie.[1] His theory is that neurotic conflicts originate in the experience of separation from the mother. It is an experience we all have to pass through and undoubtedly the manner of passing through it may have a lasting effect on character.

The infant is psychologically undifferentiated from the mother for many months after birth. The infant has been the object of solicitude and attention on the part of the mother; to her the child turns for every gratification of its needs, physical and psychological. Its discomforts, its pains, its joys, its strivings are brought to her. A brother or sister now arrives on the scene. The mother must now give a large part of her attention to the newcomer and less to the elder child. Or it may be there is no other child, but the separation from the mother is still inevitable. The wise mother knows that the child must transfer some of its interest to others outside the family; it must become independent of her. In that crisis of separation from the mother, Dr. Suttie believed that an anxiety-situation arises, and the child's reaction to the anxiety will determine the child's reaction to life in general. He gives four possible reactions:

First the child may feel that the mother does not love it any more; but it may attempt to preserve the mother's goodness and lovableness. The child will thus tend to blame itself for what it thinks is a change in the mother's love. It is as if the child said: "If mother does not love me it is because I am bad; but mother is good." This reaction will tend to set up inferiority feelings which may lead to melancholia.

Secondly, the child may through experience associate the

[1] *Origins of Love and Hate*, pages 43ff.

mother with babies and illness. The child then acts as if it said : 'Mother is kind to babies and to those who are ill." The child may then take the flight into psychological illness in order to get the mother's affection and solicitude. Pushed far enough this reaction may lead ultimately to dementia praecox, a very severe psychosis.

Thirdly, the child may repudiate its desire for the mother's love and become aggressive. It may react as if it had said : " I can get a better mother than you." Here the mother's loveableness is thrown aside as though the child thought the mother was bad and had denied it its rights. In this case the child, according to Dr. Suttie, may turn to the father who, up till this time, has been little in the picture ; he then becomes *the* parent and, to quote Suttie, " if it does not interfere with the sexual attitude of the boy, or produce excessive ' father fixation ' in the girl, it can be looked upon as normal, as it ultimately leads on to the adoption of the whole social environment in lieu of the mother ".

A fourth possibility remains open to the child. The child may seek to coerce the love of the mother. Here it is as if the child had said : " If you don't love me you will fear me." Delinquency is largely the product of this reaction.

Now there can be no doubt that separation-anxiety can play a large part in shaping a basic reaction to life ; nor can there be the slightest doubt that we meet with many people whose general reaction to life can be expressed in terms such as those Suttie has used. We all know the father or mother who compels obedience in the child by threatening to withdraw love, or to be cross ; we know the men and women who can compel their married partners to fall in with their wishes under the implicit threat of days of sulks and silence. There are others ready to threaten suicide if any wish is left ungratified. Likewise, we know people who are always blaming themselves if anything goes wrong ; and that tendency, if it becomes pathological, is seen in people who can get tremendous fear if they hear or read of someone dying or in an accident ; they worry themselves as to whether they have had anything to do with it. It is not uncommon to find people who can remember the phantasies they had in which they pictured another mother, and endowed her with all the qualities they thought their own mother did not possess. The same reaction can be seen in men and women not too happily married. They have a phantasy of the kind of man or woman they would marry if their present husband or wife died ! I took the trouble for almost two years to make a point of asking male patients if they already had chosen their second wife ! To my astonishment everyone had pictured to himself the kind of wife he would marry if given the opportunity to marry again ; and some had even seen her ! There are many people who have adopted the social environment, or who serve society whole-heartedly. But this is not necessarily a reaction to the loss of the mother.

Dr. Suttie's theory is simple, indeed, I think, too simple to explain all the character-traits we find in normal and abnormal people. The father plays a much more important part than Suttie seems to admit. Nor do I think that all our reactions are conditioned by the child's desire for the mother's love. It is probable that the reaction to authority has a deeper influence on the child's character-formation. Erich Fromm has shown that in its reaction to authority the child may become submissive in order to feel secure from the father's punishment or disapproval. The submissiveness, however, generates a rebel drive which is directed against the authoritarian parent ; and the child may become afraid of and repress the hostile feelings. Such hostility against the parent on whom we are dependent causes still more insecurity. That reaction to authority may become a habitual mode of reacting to authority in life and cause endless difficulty.

Karen Horney's investigations[1] to some extent confirm the views of Dr. Suttie. She thinks that the need for affection is a basic need in the child and indeed in the adult. The child deprived of affection or who thinks it is denied will then set up a character-structure which she calls the neurotic need for affection. The growing personality will seek by all means to be liked and approved ; it will automatically live up to the expectation of others in order to get their affection or approval. Such a person will, in all probability, generate hostile feelings within himself and become afraid of them lest they endanger his crying need, namely the affection and approval of others. Both Fromm and Karen Horney forget that the individual may remain submissive and become a " yes " person with the result that they never develop initiative or personality. She shows clearly, as does Fromm, this basic need for approval. The sociologist would say that we need recognition or status and to be accepted as one not only *in* the society but " of " the society.

I think also that the feeling of " aloneness " and isolation felt by so many people is due to the unconscious lack of security in regard to other people's love for them. There can be no question of the fact that to be loved and to love does give that sense of belonging to someone, that sense of security which is necessary to the possession of confidence. Without confidence we cannot face life. The child does tend to keep its reactions to frustrations and deprivations of early life, and they become character-structures.

What I think is forgotten by Dr. Suttie, and to some extent by both Fromm and Karen Horney, is the moral factor. The Freudians forget ethics and practically treat

---

[1] *The Neurotic Personality of Our Time* ; also *Self-Analysis.*

the individual as though he were not a moral being at all. Karen Horney calls for courage on the part of psychotherapists to deal with the neurotic's moral problems. Actually, in Suttie's theory, two of the four reactions supposed to be taken by the child at the time of separation from the mother are ethical and not merely psychological. When a child says, " If mother does not love me it is because I am bad," there is a moral judgment. Similarly when the child says the mother is bad. Personally I should be inclined to place more emphasis upon the child's reactions to its moral imperatives. With the capacity for moral experience the child comes for the first time upon guilt-feelings in the true sense of the term. My observations incline me to the view that the reaction of the child to these guilt-feelings has a decisive effect in the formation of character-structure. The case of the woman mentioned on pages 15ff is a very good example.

Here there is no question of separation from the mother causing the anxiety ; nor was there any need to be " submissive " to a threatening mother or father. The whole trouble begins and continues as a reaction to moral ideas and religious imperatives. Her reaction to guilt-feelings has been her undoing. Those guilt-feelings gave her the strong impression that she was not secure with God. That insecurity with God was repressed ; and she tries through her intellect and through her compulsive drive towards sexual unassailability to find that security and cannot. Her sexual impulses have still strong guilt associated with them in the unconscious and this is displaced upon those who are known to have committed some sexual fault. It is not beside the point to mention that the accentuation of her symptoms coincided with her daughter's marriage.

Moral security, religious assurance, the great majority of neurotic individuals ask for and need. And it seems to me

to be useless to think there can be any advance in psychotherapeutic theory until this is more widely recognized. The
threat to moral security comes from within the individual,
not from without. That would seem also to be the view
of Jung. It is religion alone that can give the requisite sense
of moral security ; but a religion of grace, not law ; of
mercy, not of judgment.

What I think we can say about the origin of conflicts is
that we cannot predicate one situation to which all conflicts
can be traced. To seek for the origin of love and hate in the
one situation of separation from the mother will make us
read theory into fact instead of taking our theories from the
observation of psychological facts themselves. No doubt
there are a number of individuals whose psychology can be
explained by their reaction to separation-anxiety ; but there
are a great number more that by no sound reasoning can
fit into the theory. So in regard to the theory of Submissiveness and Hostility of Erich Fromm. It certainly explains
many individuals' psychology, and especially the psychology
of many public leaders who show the contradictory trends
of submissiveness to authority, yet rebellion against it, and
also manifest a strong authoritarian strain in themselves.

Karen Horney has made an important contribution
comparable to Fromm's in her descriptions of the character-
trends formed in the interest of getting affection.[1] More
patients can be explained by this theory than any other, in
my opinion. This compulsive need for affection can
motivate all sorts of trends. If there is any phrase that gives
us the root of the various neuroses, however, though I doubt
if there is, it is " the need for security " ; moral security
against the uprush of our own sexual, or hostile impulses ;
economic security against the uncertainty of our economic

[1] See *The Neurotic Personality of Our Time, New Ways of
Psycho-Analysis,* and *Self-Analysis.*

order ; religious security against the actual fact of our moral frailty, reinforced by a need for a meaning to life that can help us to stand four-square against the contradictions and uncertainties of life, and which alone can help us to stand up against a ruthless prohibitive conscience.

It is possible to go to childhood and trace the origins of psychological troubles in the reaction of the child to the crises through which it has to pass. It is possible to say that the trouble arises in the unresolved conflicts of childhood which have become repressed. And certainly childhood's repressions and conflicts alone can explain the predisposition to the actual breakdown. Too much stress should not, however, be laid upon this. Education, we must remember, begins with self-consciousness ; and hence the modification of childhood's conflicts is steadily going on unless the conflicts are thoroughly repressed in childhood. Education should not be merely an organizing of the child's knowledge of the external world, nor a mere developing of the child's innate abilities ; it should be more directly focussed upon the integration of the child's natural interests, its behaviour-tendencies, and its abilities, with its moral and religious sentiments. Nor should educationists forget that the child needs to be socialized. In other words, the whole child has to be integrated with the community. Cultural standards and moral traditions should not be steel hoops into which the child must be fitted ; they must be like elastic bands, able to stretch and take in new thought ; they should leave room for ever widening moral and religious horizons. No moral, religious or social progress can be made unless we are training the children to question the tacit assumptions on which our moral, religious, economic and social order rests. The relation of our social and economic order to the failure of many to realize their personality as well as to the neuroses is too big a subject to do more than mention here. The relation, however,[1] is there and has far more to do with our troubles than many realize.

All these theories I have mentioned lay very little stress upon sex as a causative factor of character-disturbance. I think that is in the right direction. The deeper one gets into a human being the more one finds that the roots of the trouble are not sexual ; but that most of the sexual troubles are reactions to something more basic.

What conditions our reactions to situations in childhood ? Here we come upon an ultimate problem. The factor of the child's personality is one that should never be forgotten. The external or internal situation that causes the feeling of insecurity is never more than the opportunity for the child's soul to react. Even our heredity does not matter much. How do we react to our inheritance is the vital question ? One child reacts to insecurity or to a situation in one way and another in another way. No doubt in the meeting where the woman patient's troubles began there were other children who took no harm ; and no doubt they had their childish conflicts also ; but only the patient reacted in the way we know she did. The child and the adult react vitally to a situation in accordance with something we call individuality, and never mechanically. Why one should react in one way and another in another to approximately the same situation or a similar one was asked by Freud and Suttie ; but not answered. Rivers thought that education was the vital factor. It is doubtful whether an answer can be given. What we do know is that children are at first spontaneous and react through their own individuality, which is their birthright. As far as possible the parent and educator should so train the child that it will be able to keep its spontaneity. That spontaneity means freedom, or what

---

[1] Cf. *The Neurotic Personality of Our Time*, by Karen Horney, final chapter.

elsewhere I have called self-possession. The late Professor James Ward has a sentence worth remembering in this connection. " The value ", he writes, " of a single man or woman of open mind, independent judgment, and moral courage, who requires to be convinced and refuses to be cajoled, is only concerned to be right and not afraid to be singular, deferring to reason but not to rank, true to his or her own self and therefore not false to any man—the value of such a man or woman, I say, is priceless : a nation of such would leaven and regenerate the world. That is the true national education at which England should aim. What we actually aim at is something immeasurably inferior."[1]

Now I have stated these conflicts and their symptoms in pathological pictures. I have done so advisedly. My reason for doing so is that I have come to the conclusion that the problems which give rise to the lesser and grosser neurotic conflicts are not different from the problems common to us all, either in childhood or adulthood. The pathological picture gives an outsize of our own reactions. The people whose conflicts have reached the pathological stage are not as different from ourselves as we should like to think. They are different, else they would not be as they are. But it is not because they have problems different from those the ordinary child and man has to face, but because they have resorted to repression which can never give us a solution ; it simply drives the conflict within. Recall as many cases as I can, both in reading and practice, and I cannot find an instance in which one of what the Catholic Church calls the " seven deadly sins " is not repressed. Either the symptoms are the expression of the means whereby the individual is defending himself against one of the " deadly sins ", or they are the means by which he is attempting to gratify one of them without guilt.

[1] *Psychology Applied to Education*, pages 182f.

One thing we must carefully note about these character-structures which lead to personality-disturbances, and that is the capacity we have for simulating the virtues. It has been known for long that in neurotic disease the individual's repressed emotions and impulses can be expressed in physical symptoms, such as functional paralysis, acceleration of the heart's beat, high blood-pressure, asthma, etc., etc. A good diagnostician can recognize almost at once that there is an indiscriminateness about the neurotic symptoms absent entirely from the organically produced symptoms. The character-neuroses can simulate the striving for moral and spiritual ideals or can clothe itself in the garments of virtue in such a way as to deceive the very angels of heaven. The woman with a neurotic love for her husband would, at a certain stage of her trouble, pass almost for a perfect lover. She is never happy unless her husband is with her in the home or accompanying her outside. One would think that she had only one thought and that was to love and serve her husband. Her love, however, is motivated to get, not to give ; she soon reaches a stage when her demands and expectations are excessive, her anger indiscriminate ; she begins to fear going out alone, even becomes afraid of her husband going out at all, even to work. I have quoted James Ward on the value of the individual of independent mind. We get people with a neurotic urge for independence, whose urge is really the outcome of a fear of dependence, of the responsibilities of love, and a neurotic dread of any ties whatsoever. I have had a good many patients whose trouble was due to a puritanic conscience of which they were unconsciously afraid. If one took them at their face value one would think that they were motivated by moral ideals of the purest water. Actually they are trying to prove to themselves that no temptation can assail them ; they fear evil rather than hate it. Hence their pre-occupation with self-blame and avoidance of anything like sin. Their drive is negative not positive. They spend their lives guarding themselves against going down the by-ways of sin instead of getting along the highway of virtue.

Enough has been said to show that the neurotic has no drives which are not in the normal person. In the perversions the drive is directed to wrong objects, but the drive in itself towards satisfaction—e.g. sexual satisfaction—is perfectly normal. In the character-drives such as the need for affection, or independence, or the moral ideal, the motives are wrong. These are not wanted for their own sake but as protection against insecurity or against repressed impulses. Nor does the neurotic meet problems which are not common to us all. It is his manner of resolving his problems that is wrong. To some degree we are all subject to the neurotic's troubles. Is that not why there is such a widespread and general interest in abnormal psychology? Is it not because people see themselves as in a mirror, their own conflicts in an exaggerated form, their cravings and contradictions, and the needs of their own souls in what they read, that they buy so many psychological books?

Perhaps the pastor should remember this as he ascends the pulpit Sunday after Sunday. It is safe to say that there is not a single service in which many in the congregation are there because of difficulties in their own lives that need to be smoothed out; with sins which they are conscious need forgiveness; with weaknesses for which they need strength; with habits they would fain overcome. How many people in any one congregation have frustrations to which the neurotic has reacted in the wrong way! How many have brow-beating consciences that give them not a moment's peace! You cannot draw a hard and last line between neuroticism and the frailty of human flesh.

If, then, the pastor is to minister to his people he must

have a rational education in psychology. If he has that, will he not the better understand the conflicts to which his people are continually subject, and help to keep those conflicts from becoming pathological ? Will he not be prepared to help his people to meet in a rational way the complicated psychological problems of the modern man and woman ? It would seem to be part of the pastor's job to help his young people especially to recognize their conflicts, and to help them to resolve them in such a way that their needs, both biological and psychological will be integrated with the prospective aim of personality, and with the social environment in which they must live.

I think that most pastors love their work and their people ; those who do, generally have some psychological capacity for seeing into the difficulties of the soul. It needs, however, to be said that the minister cannot help his people to see and to correct the causes of their difficulties unless he first knows himself, and unless he is not afraid to look into himself and see the mental processes behind his own behaviour ; unless he is able to see the sources of his own weaknesses, as well as to recognize them. He must have his own ideal of psychological, moral and spiritual maturity. It does not follow that only the man who is himself perfectly unified is the only one able to help others who are distressed or immature. Did not St. Paul himself speak of his divided mind ? That which he wanted to do he could not do, and that which he detested doing he was compelled to do ? Did he not speak of the subtlety of sin when he said : " Sin that it might appear sin worketh death through that which is good " ? Did he not speak of not yet having apprehended that for which he had been apprehended but that he still pressed on ? Indeed, it is only as we can incipiently at least experience the conflicts in the souls of others that we are likely to be able to help them. One does not need to be an expert in psychotherapy to help people with conflicts which are not repressed ; they are the same conflicts which afflict our own souls.

In closing, let me try to sum up one or two of the principles which anyone can put into practice in his ministry. They are in reality principles of mental hygiene.

The first I have already hinted at. It is : Know yourself ; be able to see yourself in the mirror of your people's difficulties, troubles and weaknesses. That alone can give you first-hand knowledge of this branch of psychology. To know psychology through books, unless the books have been a mirror of your own soul, will only bewilder you. You must study the data of your science within yourself, the only place where you can see all the data at first hand.

It needs courage to do this ; it needs humility so that you will not look down upon yourself but ever up to God. That is why psychology is a dangerous subject. Not everyone is fitted or has the courage to see his unconscious motives, his hates and drives. I have again and again thought during my long experience of neurotic troubles that unless a man has a really grounded faith and assurance of God's grace he would be best to keep away from analysis altogether. It can offer more temptations to a man who is not sure of himself or God than any other vocation. Although I have said that sexual trouble is as a rule never the root of neurotic symptoms, there are few cases where sexual temptations and difficulties have not to be dealt with. Unless a man knows himself he is very likely to become involved personally before he is conscious of what is happening. Only recently I have dealt with a woman whose pastor I should think meant to be sympathetic but who raised a storm of passion in the woman which I have found very difficult to calm. It is here that the rational education in psychology comes to your aid. You come prepared to your task like the medical practitioner ;

like him you learn to inhibit undesirable feelings which might involve you in the patient's neurotic cravings.

The second direction is that those who would be true pastors must cultivate an intelligent sympathy and unlimited patience with human frailty, and self-delusions. If you understand your own problems, and are dealing with them faithfully, then it follows that your sympathy will be intelligent and not a blind sympathy that ends in mere feeling. It will be a sympathy that springs from knowledge, and which will keep you from becoming involved in the individual's problems. If you know yourself, you will know with what patience and long-suffering God has dealt with you, and you will never lose patience with those who come to you with their troubles.

Here are some simple rules of mental hygiene worth remembering :

1. Help your people to acquire a healthy self-criticism, and elicit in them the courage to face themselves in God's presence. Self-examination need have no dangers unless it has become a morbid introspection. In self-examination we should put ourselves as it were outside ourselves ; we should try to see ourselves objectively. My impulses are mine but they are not me ; my sins are mine but they are not me ; my mind does not consent to them. That should be the attitude you help your people to cultivate. Did not St. Paul say that it was no longer he that did wrong but the sin that dwelt in him ? Paul looked at himself not through the morbid spectacles of introspection. Introspection of a morbid kind is ever looking for flaws ; self-examination looks so as to better oneself.[1]

2. Help your people to stop crying for what they cannot get. In other words, you must help them to adjust to their frustrations in so far as these cannot be removed. There are

[1] See note at end of lecture.

frustrations which cannot be avoided. Every childless woman suffers frustration ; everyone whose innate abilities have never had the chance to be exercised because of a lack of education suffers frustration. Death, as a rule, means the frustration of love for someone.

3. Help your people to see as scientific fact that what matters for mental and spiritual health is not what happens to them, nor what they have done, nor what behaviour-tendencies are recognized within themselves, but how they react to them all. It is our response that creates the psychological situation, not the mere external circumstances or the solicitation of our behaviour-tendencies.[1]

4. Help them to accept as a scientific fact that religion is not an optional activity we can indulge or leave alone ; but a foundation of life, that on which a strong life stands secure and is never alone. To find religion is to find what life means for us ; it is not merely to be adjusted to life and to the demands of our nature, but to be reconciled to God and to life. It is one thing to get a meaning to life and another to yield ourselves to it ; it is one thing to have religion and another to have a spontaneous relation to it. The pessimist has a meaning to life ; but it is doubtful if he is reconciled to it. He may defy life because of his pessimistic philosophy, and mistake defiance for reconciliation, as McDougall does in his *Character, Conduct and Life*. Henley's poem about the head that is bloody but unbowed is not reconciliation, but a hurling of defiance at the worst life can do. He has found no meaning to life, all he can do is to hurl defiance at it.

5. There is one far-reaching principle in psychotherapy, according to Dr. McCurdy. In his own words it is this : " If a man has courage, he may learn to triumph over almost every mental abnormality with the aid of psychological

[1] See note at end of lecture.

knowledge. Without it, his only hope lies in his environment being altered to suit his weakness."[1]

I myself would add "faith" to "courage", although we must remember that courage is an outward expression of faith.

These are simple rules of mental hygiene, but they are not to be despised because of that. They are within the reach of everyone. The rules of physical hygiene are just as simple : fresh air, decent food and sleep, good sanitation and some physical exercise. Through these simple rules of hygiene we may acquire a spontaneous relation to our human nature, to our fellow man and to God. In the spontaneity of our relations lies our mental health.

It will not be out of place here to remember that behind all rules there should be a clearer idea as to what is meant by a mature adult.[2] After all it is the failure to reach maturity that is manifested in our weaknesses, our neurotic symptoms, our hasty tempers, and our "all or nothing" reactions to life.

Economic maturity is the sign that a man is able to maintain himself without having to resort to some form of parasitism. Given the chance, the economically mature adult will not only maintain himself but will make his economic contribution to the society which gives him the economic and moral means of life. Work is a foundation of life as of society.

When an individual is mature there is a natural urge to fall in love and to marry and have children. This maturity is much more difficult to reach than ordinary people realize. Many people can fall in love but when it comes to getting married they break down. Some can get married but for

[1] *Psychology of Emotion*, page 441.
[2] Cf. *The Psychology of the Adolescent*, by Leta S. Hollingworth, Chapter VIII.

psychological reasons they are unable to perform the act that brings children. This biological maturity includes the capacity for spontaneous sexual relations in which both partners are able to get full physical and psychological satisfaction from coitus. It is astonishing the large percentage of women especially who never reach a climax in these marital relations. When such is the case there is apt to be manifested nervous symptoms.

We have already spoken about the effects of submissiveness. We can submit to political or religious dogma without ever finding grounds in our own thinking for the views that we hold. The intellectually mature adult arrives at his opinion by "original thought", as Erich Fromm puts it. This does not mean that he finds new truth. His opinions may not be different from that of his father, his class or his Church ; but they are "original" in the sense that they are grounded in his own thought. The result is that his views are not likely to crash when he comes up against the contradictions of life. If they are original in the sense we have used the term, they will hold the individual firm ; and they will be able to expand with widening experience. It is beliefs we hold at second-hand that crash ; first-hand beliefs change and develop but do not let us down.

There is no capacity which shows the mature adult better than the capacity to transfer our interests from the objects which were perfectly legitimate at one period of life, to the objects and responsibilities of the next period. That is always the capacity of the psychologically mature adult. I have seen a great many men and women whose symptoms were the outcome of the fact that they really had not left behind the interests which are natural in a person who is single, for the interests which ought to be primary in a married man or woman. The ego-centric interests of the adolescent "on the make" must be transferred to his responsibilities to the community if he is to grow up and become mature. In other words, he has to develop socialized interests. There are individuals who tend to become fixated on early objects such as the parents, or it may be upon early infantile habits. It is these that often lead to distressing neurotic trouble. The psychologically mature adult is self-possessed ; his mental processes are under his control to send them where he wishes. His mental processes and drives are his servants ; they are directed by adult demands and adult ends.

Spiritual maturity is not very easy to define ; but that it is one of the necessities has been implied throughout these lectures. No man can be said to have reached maturity who has not found some meaning to life. Often I have thought of spiritual maturity and tried to define it. One thing is certain, it is not determined by dogma, although it is no enemy of dogma in the true sense of that much abused term. The older I grow and the more I ask the question, " In what does spiritual maturity consist ? " I am led back to the Shorter Catechism and to an answer I must often have repeated before I had the slightest idea of its meaning. It is the answer to the profoundest question we can ask : " What is the chief end of man ? " To me the Shorter Catechism gives the most satisfying answer : *" The chief end of man is to glorify God and to enjoy Him for ever."* Curiously enough, although the chief design of the catechism is to put beliefs into children's minds it does not say that the chief end of man is to believe in Him, but " to enjoy Him ". To enjoy God—that is the only way in which we can glorify God. From the psychological point of view at least, the enjoyment of God is religion. Religion, like art, is an enjoyment ; an experience of joy. As the lover of art enjoys beauty, so the lover of God enjoys religion. It is the real psychological test of spiritual maturity. The man who is the victim of an unhappy holiness is immature. A holy happiness, an enjoyment of God, is the mark of adulthood in religion.

These, then, are the marks of the individual who is mature. Such a man is likely to be adjusted to his own nature and the demands of social life. He may, however, be mature in some aspects of his nature and in others still infantile or adolescent. To the extent he is not mature he will be unadjusted if not maladjusted to life.

These marks of adulthood the pastor should look for in himself. It is a commonplace of psychotherapy that patients endow the analyst with all the virtues and qualities they themselves lack. To a very great degree he becomes the picture of the unified self, the mature individual they are themselves seeking to be. It is not an erotic phenomenon as Freud thought, although it may become so in the hands of a careless analyst. It is the so-called "transference". It becomes the basis of faith in the analyst; and the skilful analyst or pastor uses it to overcome all the hindrances to adulthood. The people we can help by way of spiritual direction and an opening of their eyes until they see themselves will intuit in us the qualities they are lacking yet longing to acquire, and for lack of which they are distressed in mind or spirit. If people need faith to grope in the dark, will not our personal faith elicit the intuition of faith in them ? If they have confused lust with love will they not recognize the difference in our happiness and fidelity ? If they have been disillusioned by the world and have no hope, will not their hope revive when they see that disillusionment for you has not deprived you of hope, but deepened it because it has led to a stronger staying of the mind on God ?

NOTE TO LECTURE 4

MR. NEWSHAM, in the course of reading through the typescript, has asked two questions relative to the principles of treatment I have given in the fourth lecture. He thinks there is something contradictory in the contention throughout the lectures that we must accept ourselves, and the contention of this section that we must realize that my "impulses are mine but not 'me'". He says: "But I thought it imperative that I must realize that I am this sort of person; that it is myself who is lustful, envious, proud."

There is no contradiction. We must differentiate within the self two centres from which we can react. There is the *ego*, that centre round which there has been organized our tendencies to react to whatever solicits the *ego*. In other words, the *ego* is that centre of reaction that is moved wholly by inclination, and the inclinations are characterized by pleasure and pain. On the other hand, there is the subject that is moved by will, and the movements of the will are characterized by rationality. The *ego* moves according to the principle of pleasure-pain, and is dominated by the strongest inclination. The real self, the self as a whole, does not ask whether an inclination is pleasurable or painful; it simply asks whether the inclination is good or bad, false or true, just or unjust. In the neurotic this self plays a very little part; the *ego* is controlled by the infantile prohibitive conscience and is thus coerced by fear. The real self cannot be coerced (cf. quotation from James Ward in this lecture). When Professor Laird[1] says: "the sentiments being only certain systems of inclinations and solicitations, do not govern. When we follow or reject them with our might, and in the teeth of adversity, because of our belief that we ought to do

[1] *A Study in Moral Theory*, page 138.

so, we have a plain example of this truth ", he is really implying that the solicitations which we reject, or the inclinations we follow in the teeth of adversity are rejected or accepted by the self in spite of the ego. The self or subject is the final arbiter.

Hence, when I say " my impulses are mine but not me ", I mean that I am conscious of inclinations and solicitations which are alien to my sense of the rational and moral, and the self rejects them. In the example of the woman who, when she dreamed something she did not like, said that it came from my patient and not from her, she was really right in one sense that the dreams were alien to her rational and moral self. Her fault lay in the fact that she did not realize that there were tendencies in her psychological make-up which would solicit her *ego* but could not be repudiated by the self because they were unconscious and only came up in dreams. She had to accept the fact that they came from her mind.

There is a real need for the study of the psychological analysis of the whole self or individual. In philosophy we are familiar with the distinction between the empirical ego and the transcendental ego. This distinction is psychological terms is the *ego* moved by inclination and the self moved by rationality. Whether this " horizontal " division of the individual can be justified is a question too large to be considered here.

The second point raised by Mr. Newsham is the contention in the lecture that it is our reactions that matter and not the solicitations. " Isn't the basic trouble ", he asks, " the fact that how we react *is* one of our behaviour-tendencies ? What when a man deplores how he reacts as much as anything ? Can we give hope to such a man ? Can Christ redirect his reaction behaviour ?

This is a relevant question. What was in my mind,

however, was the fact that so many get panic-stricken by the very presence of solicitations alien to the moral ideals in their conscious mind that unconsciously they tend to repress them. Once the individual realizes that he need not be afraid of the solicitations, and that he cannot help them coming into his mind, his reactions come within his control. He knows he could go to the devil in an hour but that he needn't and wouldn't. Here his religion comes to him as power to react in such a way as to modify as well as to withstand the solicitations. The classical passage is the seventh chapter of Romans, where Paul, speaking of his inability to do what he ought to do, cries: " Who shall deliver me from the body of this death ? I thank Thee through our Lord Jesus Christ." And again: " I can do all things through Christ who strengtheneth me " (Phil. iv. 13). Dr. Dodd, in his commentary on Romans, contends that this seventh chapter is an account of Paul's behaviour-tendencies previous to conversion. If that contention is correct, then Paul had found that Christ could determine his reactions to evil solicitations.